Eat, Fast, Feast

EAT, FAST, FEAST

Heal Your Body While Feeding Your Soul—
A Christian Guide to Fasting

Jay W. Richards

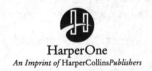

HarperOne
An Imprint of HarperCollinsPublishers

HarperOne

EAT, FAST, FEAST. Copyright © 2020 by Jay W. Richards. All rights
reserved. Printed in the United States of America. No part of
this book may be used or reproduced in any manner whatsoever
without written permission except in the case of brief quotations
embodied in critical articles and reviews. For information, address
HarperCollins Publishers, 195 Broadway, New York, NY 10007.

HarperCollins books may be purchased for educational, business,
or sales promotional use. For information, please email the
Special Markets Department at SPsales@harpercollins.com.

FIRST EDITION

Designed by Diahann Sturge

Library of Congress Cataloging-in-Publication
Data is available upon request.

ISBN 978-0-06-290521-5

20 21 22 23 24 LSC 10 9 8 7 6 5 4 3 2 1

In memory of my mother, Josephine Richards
September 14, 1943–December 13, 2018

CONTENTS

Week Four

Week Five

Week Six

The Physician Within

We've spent decades debating what we ought to eat. Should we eat bread? Should we eat butter? Should we eat a low-fat diet? Should we eat a high-fat diet? The combinations are endless and the advice ever-changing. Despite this often-misguided fixation on what to eat, we spend little time studying another, just as crucial question: *when* to eat. Based on a paucity of scientific debate, many of us have been advised by "experts" to eat early and often. The idea that there are times when we should abstain from eating has been a minority view, to say the least. This is especially strange since fasting is one of the oldest health remedies in history. It has been part of the practice of virtually every culture on earth. Every major religion—Christianity, Judaism, Islam, Buddhism, and Hinduism—incorporates fasting into its practices. And yet rigorous fasting has virtually disappeared from modern life.

To be clear, fasting is not starvation. Fasting is the voluntary abstinence from food for spiritual, health, or other reasons. One may fast for any period of time, from a few hours to a few months. As a healing tradition, fasting has a long history. Hippocrates of Kos (c. 460–c. 370 BC), widely considered the father of modern medicine, wrote, "To eat when you are sick is to feed your illness." The ancient Greek writer and historian Plutarch (c. AD 46–c. AD 120) echoed these sentiments, advising, "Instead of using medicine, better fast today." Plato and Aristotle were also staunch supporters of fasting. Yet few who study their works today in search of wisdom follow these Greek philosophers' advice on fasting.

The ancient Greeks believed that medical treatment could be discovered by observing nature. Humans, like most animals, don't eat when they become sick. Just think of the last time you were sick with the flu. Probably the last thing you wanted to do was eat. Fasting seems to be a universal human response to all manner of illness. It's ingrained in our human heritage, as old as humankind itself. Fasting is, in that sense, instinct.

The ancient Greeks also believed that fasting improved mental clarity. Again, our common experience bears this out. Think about the last time you ate a huge Thanksgiving meal. Did you feel more energetic and mentally alert afterward? Or instead, did you feel sleepy and a little dopey? Probably the latter. That huge influx of food rerouted blood to your digestive system, leaving less blood for brain function. Fasting does the opposite, leaving more blood for your brain.

Other intellectual giants were also great champions of fasting. Take Paracelsus (1493–1541), the founder of toxicology and one of three fathers of modern Western medicine (along with Hippocrates and Galen). "Fasting is the greatest remedy," he wrote; "the physician within." Benjamin Franklin (1706–1790), one of America's founding fathers and renowned for wide knowledge, once wrote, "The best of all medicines is resting and fasting."

Fasting for spiritual purposes is widely practiced in many

parts of the world. It remains part of virtually every major religion. Jesus Christ, Buddha, and the prophet Muhammad all shared a common belief in the power of fasting. The practice of fasting developed independently among different religions and cultures, not as something that was harmful, but something that was deeply helpful to the human body and spirit.

Many Buddhists consume food only in the morning, and then fast daily from noon until the next morning. Buddhists may also undergo the rigors of various water-only fasts for days or weeks on end. Many Eastern Orthodox Christians follow various fasts over 180 to 200 days of the year. Dr. Ancel Keys, the famous nutritional researcher, often considered Crete the poster child for the healthy Mediterranean diet. One key factor may have been that Cretans followed the Greek Orthodox tradition of fasting.

Muslims fast from sunrise to sunset during the month of Ramadan. The prophet Muhammad also encouraged fasting every week on Mondays and Thursdays. Ramadan differs from most fasting protocols since fluids as well as foods are forbidden. Further, since eating is permitted before sunrise and after sunset, recent studies indicate that daily caloric intake actually rises a lot during this period. Gorging before sunrise and after sunset, especially on highly refined carbohydrates, negates much of fasting's benefit.

Many people assume these are just outdated folk and religious traditions that have no basis in science. But the truth is just the opposite. There is now a mountain of scientific and clinical evidence that fasting is good for us, and that it may be the cure for the so-called diseases of civilization that afflict so many modern people.

Most North Americans subsist on sugar (glucose) for energy. Our bodies can run on glucose and fat but they tend to use glucose whenever it's available. When the supply of sugar is cut off, the body, once it uses up its stored sugar (glycogen), switches to burning fat—either from the diet or from the body. Unfortunately, constant infusions of sugar in our diet keep our insulin levels high. Insulin is an important hormone that, in the presence of blood sugar, signals to the body to burn sugar and store any extra as body fat. And, to judge from the latest health statistics, we're storing more and more fat, and harming our health in the process.

Fasting strikes at the root of this problem. Done right, fasting lowers our insulin levels and helps reset our metabolism, without any harm to our health. Different lengths of fasts have different effects, but the basic idea is to deplete your body's stored sugars until it starts burning fat. Some parts of your body, such as the brain, still need some glucose but mostly use an alternate fuel, ketones, which are made from body fat. Strictly speaking, there are no essential carbohydrates.

But won't fasting slow down your metabolism and deplete your muscles? No, it won't. In the early days of a fast, your body actually *increases* its energy expenditures and protects lean mass through various hormonal signals.

But won't you be crazy hungry and get hungrier and hungrier the longer you fast? No. Fasters are often less hungry after several days without food than they were at the beginning, no doubt because their bodies are efficiently using body fat for all their energy needs.

The effects of fasting, in other words, are just the opposite of the persistent calorie reduction of long-term "diets," which rarely work in the long run. What makes fasting different from dieting is its *intermittent* nature. Diets fail because of their constancy. The defining characteristic of life on Earth is homeostasis, wherein competing processes balance out in a state of equilibrium. In the body, any constant stimulus will eventually be met with an adaptation. With persistent calorie reduction, the body at some point responds by reducing total energy expenditure. This leads to the dreaded plateau in weight loss and eventually to weight gain. Several recent studies have confirmed this.

We have spent decades obsessing over the question of what to eat, but we have virtually ignored the crucial aspect of meal timing. Weight gain is not a uniform process. Average yearly weight gain in North Americans is about 1.3 pounds per year (0.6 kilograms), but that increase is not constant. The year-end holiday period produces a whopping 60 percent of this yearly weight gain in just six weeks. Most people then lose some weight after the holidays, but not enough to counter the gain. The long-term effect, of course, is that we get fatter and fatter.

We should not always be eating, and we should not always be fasting. Feasting must be followed by fasting. When we remove the fasting and keep the feasting, we eventually get fat and sick.

Balance is the ancient secret to a long and flourishing life. Fasting follows feasting. Feasting follows fasting. Our eating must be *intermittent*, not steady. Food is a celebration of life. Every single culture in the world celebrates with large feasts. That's normal, and it's good. But religions have always reminded us that we must balance our feasting with fasting—time of "atonement," "repentance," or "cleansing." These ideas are ancient and time-tested. Should you eat lots of food on your birthday? Absolutely. Should you eat lots of food at a wedding? Absolutely. These are times to celebrate and indulge. But there is also a time to fast. We cannot feast all the time. We cannot fast all the time. It won't work. It doesn't work.

You may fear the prospect of fasting if you've never made it part of your lifestyle. So it's good to remember how common it is. There are an estimated 1.6 billion Muslims in the world, who are supposed to fast for the month of Ramadan and two days a week throughout the year. There are about 14 million Mormons, who are supposed to fast once a month. There are some 350 million Buddhists in the world, many of whom fast regularly. So, right there, almost one-third of the entire world population is supposed to routinely fast throughout their lives.

So, clearly, it can be done. Moreover, there are no lasting negative side effects to regular fasting. Quite the contrary. It appears to have extraordinary health benefits. Fasting is a cornerstone of our practice at the Intensive Dietary Management clinic in Toronto. We are using doctor-supervised fasts of shorter and longer duration to treat obesity, type 2 diabetes, and other conditions. The results are astounding. I can't believe it's not already a global protocol.

But what about those two billion Christians I didn't mention above? As Jay Richards describes in the following pages, fasting (and feasting) has been a major Christian discipline since the very beginning. Jesus fasted. The apostles fasted. Early Christians fasted. The Church Fathers and all the greatest saints have treated fasting as the natural companion to prayer.

But in the last few centuries, Christian fasts have fallen on hard times outside of the Eastern Orthodox and Eastern Rite traditions. Catholics, as Richards explains, retain vestigial fasts that often amount to going an hour without food, or avoiding certain kinds of meat on some Fridays. Some Protestants fast, but few do so consistently. I'm convinced this has had a bad effect of the health of millions of people. Richards suggests it has also harmed Christians morally and spiritually.

My expertise and experience are in physical rather than spiritual health. Our Intensive Dietary Management Program (www.idmprogram.com) offers the education and community support necessary to successfully implement fasting into your life. But I have hoped that someone would write a book on the spiritual benefits of fasting that takes account of the growing scientific and clinical evidence for its benefits to health. I'm pleased that Jay Richards has woven together the Christian tradition's rich teaching and practice with the growing scientific case for fasting. Almost anyone can benefit from fasting, but Christians have many good reasons to make it a permanent part of their lifestyle.

—Jason Fung, MD
September 2019

Jason Fung, MD, is a nephrologist, founder of the Intensive Dietary Management Program—which provides a unique treatment focus for type 2 diabetes and obesity—and author of *The Obesity Code* and *The Diabetes Code*.

INTRODUCTION

Fasting gives birth to prophets and strengthens the power-
ful; fasting makes lawgivers wise. Fasting is a good safe-
guard for the soul, a steadfast companion for the body, a
weapon for the valiant, and a gymnasium for athletes. Fast-
ing repels temptations, anoints unto piety; it is the comrade
of watchfulness and the artificer of chastity. In war it fights
bravely, in peace it teaches stillness.

—St. Basil the Great

Christians used to fast. A lot. It was a basic part of life, like eating, sleeping, working, feasting, and praying. Fasting allowed Christians to identify with Christ's suffering, to enrich their prayer life, to help feed the poor, to seek God's will, to discipline their wills, to grow in holiness, to prepare for spiritual warfare, even to battle demons.

Over the centuries, the Church developed fasting days and fasting seasons, punctuated by feast days when they would celebrate God's blessings. Think Advent followed by Christmas, and Lent followed by Easter. A careful outsider observer circa AD 600 would have noted that Christians ate modestly on most days; ate little or nothing on Wednesdays and Fridays; and feasted on Sundays. He would have noticed the same threefold pattern repeated on different dates and timescales that would not be easy to decipher from the outside.

This pattern of eating, fasting, and feasting defined the life of Christians for most of the Church's history. It lingers faintly in our language and our customs. We call the first meal of the day break*fast*. We give up something for Lent. Catholics eat less on Ash Wednesday and Good Friday and avoid meat on Fridays during Lent.

In other words, now, for the most part, we don't fast. Not really. At least not in the West. We have settled into mere vestigial fasting.

What happened?

For one thing, we're a pampered lot compared to our ancestors. Most of us have never gone a full day without eating. We get shaky if we go more than four hours without a vanilla latte or yogurt smoothie or granola bar or protein shake.

Our abundance has allowed us to be more gluttonous and slothful than our ancestors. In the developed world, no one really fears starvation. Few of us even experience food shortages. So we have less reason to eat small portions than our great-grandparents did. In fact, processed foods are so cheap that obesity is more often a disease of the poor than the rich.

Still, that's only a small part of the story. After all, most Americans have enjoyed a food bounty for a century. Yet obesity and type 2 diabetes have spiked only in the last forty years or so.

And these diseases don't track simply with gluttony and sloth. Imagine you see an obese woman and a thin man in a restaurant. The woman is eating a plate of spaghetti with a side of breadsticks. The thin man is eating a chicken breast with a side salad. Seems simple, right? The woman is a glutton.

Simple or not, you won't be able to tell from this scene which, if either, is really a glutton. You might assume the woman is fat *because* she lacks self-control and eats too much. But perhaps, for complex reasons we'll discuss later, her body partitions the energy from her food as body fat, leaving precious little for her to use for vigorous exercise. She's not fat because she eats so much. She eats so much because she's fat. She's fat, for the most part, through no fault of her own. The man, in contrast, converts most of what he eats to useful energy, so he doesn't need to eat a lot to feel full and go about his daily business.

What's absurd is that many of us eat the way we do because officials have said it's good for us. Better research has turned this idea on its head, but most people have heard little about our new knowledge. Instead, we've heard a drumbeat of "sciency" arguments proclaiming that we should avoid fat and consume lots of grains and other carbs. You know the pasta and breadsticks the overweight woman at the restaurant is eating? She may very well be following the advice of the USDA and the American Heart Association.

I lived and preached this false gospel for years. As a strength and fitness trainer in college, I even encouraged overweight fellow students to avoid obesifying fat and eat lots of "complex" carbs such as whole wheat. It seemed like simple math: One gram of fat packs nine calories, while a gram of carbohydrate or protein has only four calories. So, if you want to lose body fat, you should stay away from fat in your diet.

We're also told to eat lots of small meals throughout the day. This habit, we think, keeps our arteries clear, our blood sugar steady, and our body from going into starvation mode, where it clings to fat and sheds muscle. It also keeps us from getting famished and bingeing on Little Debbie Snack Cakes, we're told. I couldn't count the number of fitness articles I've read over the years touting this line. I spent years prompting my daughters to eat breakfast as soon as they got out of bed, based on this advice.

Even those untutored in these bogus fitness arguments are now locked into the grazing habit. It's just what we do—as natural as breathing. We wouldn't dream of telling our kids, as parents did for most of the twentieth century, to eat only three meals a day with no snacks between. Does anyone still worry about spoiling their appetite? We act as if people had always had treats at 10:00 a.m. and 2:00 p.m. and scarfed down a big bowl of Wheaties right before bed. And if other folks don't do that, isn't that just too bad for them? Why would we give up these habits if we don't need to?

At a recent conference I attended, the daily food routine went like this: hearty American breakfast buffet at 8:00 a.m.; pastries, fruit, and coffee at 10:30 a.m.; lunch with dessert at 12:30 p.m.; cookies, popcorn, and Häagen-Dazs ice-cream bars at 3:30 p.m.; reception with drinks and hors d'oeuvres at 6:00 p.m.; dinner with dessert at 7:00 p.m.; drinks and a snack reception at 9:00 p.m. And then the next morning, the cycle started over again. I'm getting an insulin spike just thinking about it.

This grazing—that is, eating early, late, and often—is one reason we now have such a hard time fasting. If you've spent years dutifully nurturing a habit, it's hard to break it. Do you eat a meal or snack every two to four hours when you're awake? If so, every cell and organ in your body will conspire to remind you if you try to go half the day without so much as a Wheat Thin. In effect, we've trained ourselves to make fasting hard to do. That's the bad news.

The good news is that the grazing custom is only a few decades old. There's no valid reason we need to keep doing it until the Lord returns in glory. On the contrary, *science is validating the ancient Christian practice of regular, and sometimes intense, fasting.* Fasting, it turns out, is actually good for us.

Our Modern Diet Makes It Much Harder to Fast

One problem is how often we eat. The other is what we can call the SAD (standard American diet), which is not, alas, limited to the US of A. I don't just mean our actual diets, which are packed with processed carbs and refined sugar. I mean the "healthy" diet, which officially smart groups have pushed for decades. No doubt you learned, as I did, to steer clear of dietary salt and fat to protect your heart and arteries. Especially saturated fat.

The USDA's food pyramid, with carby grains at the wide bottom and fats at the tiny top, is burned into our long-term memories.[1] In recent years, the government has used a forgettable plate rather than a pyramid to explain its Dietary Guidelines for Americans.[2] These distract us from asking the obvious question: Why do we take dietary advice from a government agency that was founded to promote and subsidize the food and sugar industries? Just posing the question should help break the spell it has over us.

The result, in any case, is that we mostly run not on fat but on sugar and other carbs that turn into sugar. If we go too long without eating, we'll be ravenously hungry and overeat as soon as we gain access to the fridge or manage to pierce that tamper-proof bag of Fritos. You might think you don't eat much sugar.

Maybe you avoid Froot Loops, Twinkies, and sugary soft drinks? That's good. But if you get most of your calories from grains, then you're still running on sugar, since that's what these foods become almost as soon as they pass down your throat. Some even start to transition in your mouth.

Constant grazing and a diet high in sugar and processed carbs is a very recent trend. For millennia, people ate mostly foods that were only lightly processed. They *fasted* on some days. They ate moderately on most days—two or three meals without snacks in between. And they *feasted* just a few days a year. For much of this time, the restraint was a matter of necessity. Later, the pattern became a spiritual practice for every major religion, including Christianity. Our calendar still shows signs of this lost tradition.

Now we eat our fill every day, offering our bloodstreams a constant stream of sugar. Then on holidays ("holy days") we feast—or rather, overeat. Is it any wonder there's a growing epidemic of obesity? Already there are some one and a half billion obese people on earth, concentrated in those places most likely to eat the standard American diet.[3] At the same time there's an explosion in these same places of type 2 diabetes, Alzheimer's (which some refer to as type 3 diabetes), and other metabolic diseases.

So Why Didn't Jesus Command Us to Fast?

It's no wonder, then, that we think fasting is a bit crazy. Maybe it's okay for some desert hermits and ascetics like St. Francis of Assisi and St. Catherine of Siena. But c'mon. Jesus told us to carry our cross, not look for ways to die. How can making ourselves

crazy hungry turn our minds toward Jesus? Who gains the be-
atific vision while on Weight Watchers?

Fair enough. But these complaints often hide an argument
against fasting that is as common as it is bad: If God wants us
to fast, why didn't Jesus command us to do so? Well, the answer
is simple: because he assumed that his followers would fast. In
a chapter of Matthew that follows Jesus's forty-day fast, Jesus
speaks to the crowds in his Sermon on the Mount. He tells them
that God cares about what we do, and also why we do it. "When
you give alms," for instance, you should try to do it discreetly,
rather than seeking credit for it. "When you pray," do it privately
rather than trying to get attention. "And when you fast, do not
look dismal, like the hypocrites, for they disfigure their faces
that their fasting may be seen by men" (Matt. 5:16).

You see? Jesus took it for granted that his followers would
give alms, pray, and fast. He didn't bother to command the obvious. He focused instead on explaining how best to do all three.
Just because we can think of bad ways to fast doesn't mean we
shouldn't be doing it.

So, why don't most Christians fast? Catholics, for our part,
think we do. We abstain from some foods on fixed dates—Ash
Wednesday and Fridays during Lent, and for an hour before Communion. (We call that hour fasting!) In the past, many Protestants
avoided fasting on principle. They thought it smacked of works-
righteousness and popery—a kind of gateway drug to incense and
funny hats. In recent decades, though, evangelical authors such
as Richard Foster, author of *Celebration of Discipline*, have sought
to recover for Protestants this ancient Christian discipline.

This development has helped lay the groundwork for
some prominent fasting movements in evangelical circles. I

still remember Bill Bright's inspired crusade for a forty-day fast in the 1990s. More recently, Pastor Rick Warren discovered the breakthroughs that come with fasting and has promoted the practice at Saddleback Church in California. Unfortunately, these campaigns tend to start with a bang and end with a whimper. The general rule still holds: some Protestants fast, but it's not a large group effort anchored in the Christian calendar.

If most Christians view real fasting as weird, unimportant, legalistic, optional, or even unhealthy, we won't make it part of our lives, and we will never enjoy the blessings—physical, mental, and spiritual—that it offers. We need a paradigm shift.

Science Is Validating This Ancient Christian Practice

There are rumblings of just such a shift. A growing number of renegade physicians, scientists, and enthusiasts have started to extol the benefits of dietary fat and fasting. There are now pockets of resistance to the official wisdom of the food pyramid. Millions of people have begun to spurn the food pyramid to pursue low-carb, ketogenic, paleo, and primal diets, reporting great results. They gather by the thousands on cruises, at conferences, and in chat rooms to share low-carb recipes and fat-loss stories. Spend much time in these places, and you'll find the zeal—and imbalance—of an army of new religious converts.

While it can be hard to sift sound science from pseudoscience, more and more serious scientists and physicians defend this rebellion against both grazing and the American cult of refined grain and sugars. This body of experts argues that diets with plenty of natural fat *as well as* fasting are not only safe but far better than our modern way of eating. The combination, unlike mere calorie-restricted diets, helps us burn fat, retain muscle, stabilize our moods, and think more clearly. It can reverse diseases such as type 2 diabetes and obesity, and may even help prevent and treat Alzheimer's, Parkinson's disease, and some kinds of cancer.

These aren't just conjectures. In the peer-reviewed scientific literature there is now a staggering amount of evidence in support of fasting, with far more to come. Word is starting to leak out, so much so that fasting has quickly gone from the fringes to the fashionable. In April 2019, for instance, Twitter CEO Jack Dorsey revealed that he typically eats just one (large) meal a day and fasts from Friday evening to Sunday. A few years earlier, the press would have treated his routine as bizarre. But in 2019, *Page Six* deemed it merely "extreme."[4] The reporter warned readers that "experts typically recommended three solid meals per day or six smaller meals throughout the day."

Given our two-thousand-year history of fasting, and our belief in the unity of body and soul, Christians should be at the vanguard of this movement, not making excuses or playing catch-up.

Why This Book?

There are dozens of books that extol the benefits of either fasting, high-fat/low-carb diets, or some blend of both. In a parallel universe, there are plenty of evangelical books that extol the spiritual benefits of fasting—a deeper prayer life, victory over sin, renewal of church community, and the like.

Then, over yonder, there are some Catholic books that argue

we should fast as a sacrifice. Some Catholic authors do so half-heartedly, for fear that someone will think they're calling for the bad old days before Vatican II, when Catholics were legalistic and supposedly lacked a personal relationship with Jesus. For instance, in his book *The Spirituality of Fasting*, Msgr. Charles Murphy "sharply delineates" what he calls "dieting and supervised fasts" from "the religious practice of fasting."[5] He's right that we should fast for wholesome spiritual reasons. It doesn't follow, though, that we must ignore the other reasons, and set them at odds with the spirit.

In my research and self-experimenting, I was surprised to find little that synthesizes these threads for Christians. There's a void where books linking body and soul should exist. This is my effort to help fill the void.

In what follows, I'll explain the growing scientific evidence for what I call the fasting lifestyle. I will tout the physical, cognitive, and spiritual *benefits* of fasting (and feasting). I will argue that we should be "metabolically flexible"—which means we can easily switch our bodies from sugar-burning to fat-burning and back again. And I will challenge the misguided notion that anyone who fasts for proper spiritual reasons should not seek mental and physical benefits. This makes no sense. If we are unities of body and soul, of the dust of the earth and the breath of God, then we should assume that if fasting is good for us, then it's good for us overall—body, mind, and soul.

Spiritual Hunger

I didn't set out to write a book on this subject. I started studying and experimenting with fasting out of curiosity. Later, I started writing articles and speaking on the subject. Then, at once, both online strangers and personal acquaintances began asking me to write a book. When I spoke to Christian groups on diet and fasting, I would get mobbed with questions afterward. When I did radio interviews on the subject, callers jammed the studio lines. There was giddiness and excitement. But I often heard stories of struggle with obesity and bad health. My guess is that in the wider culture, fasting has moved from the fringes to the (almost) fashionable. Thoughtful Christians have noticed, but don't yet have many resources they can trust.

In fact, many books and websites that promote fasting and ketogenic and ancestral diets are not Christian-friendly. Many assume that humans evolved from simpler life through a blind process of natural selection sifting random mutations. They treat this as an all-purpose explanation and miss the evidence of purpose in nature. Then these authors attach to their Darwinian outlook some conjectures about the dietary habits of early humans and even non-human ancestors. They rightly call out the standard American diet. But their accounts are blind to the manifest ways God fitted the human form to thrive in a host of different ecosystems and diets, as we would expect of a Creator who called us to multiply and fill the whole earth.

Other books in this area are New Age. They often extol the merits of, say, meditation, but rarely mention prayer, even though most Americans—indeed, most humans—pray rather than meditate. Some of these books also make an idol of the dieting lifestyle they champion. We should instead want to get food off the throne of our lives, and into its proper place, where it can serve as a blessing rather than a curse. We should reconnect with food's spiritual nuances—nuances that were evident to Christians for most of our history but have been lost amid our modern abundance.

I've had Christians whisper to me that they discovered therapeutic fasting from a New Age naturopathic doctor. They feel great and wonder why the Church is behind rather than ahead of the curve on these questions. I wonder that too.

Even Nordic neo-pagan themes are starting to crop up. It's no wonder that some Christians ask, in online discussions, how to reconcile their faith with, say, the paleo diet.[6]

It's not a silly question. Didn't Jesus elevate bread and wine to sacraments and pray for our daily bread in the prayer he taught his disciples? Didn't God give the Israelites manna in the wilderness—a sort of bread—and only grudgingly add quail to the diet after they complained? Given all this, how can carbs be a problem?

First, we can assume that the manna God provided the Israelites was healthy—literally a miracle food. And as for the bread and wine of Christian history and practice, nothing about it requires the standard American diet with its sugar and industrially refined grains. The typical bread eaten at the time of Jesus was different and less refined, and therefore broke down into sugars much more gradually in the body.[7] Moreover, people ate bread at fixed times, and did not graze on it throughout the day. Add all this up, and you have a diet very different from today's SAD, even among the ancient poor who for economic reasons had to eat more bread than might have been ideal.

And keep in mind, cycles of fasting and feasting are central to the Christian tradition. If we modern-day Christians are not fasting, that means *we're* the outliers.

The Fasting Lifestyle

In the following pages, I hope to convince you that our modern diet locks us into a metabolic trap that makes fasting futile and empties our feasts of meaning. Indeed, it prevents modern Christians from having proper fasts and feasts—and from discovering their power for body, mind, and soul. Grazing six or more times a day, eating lots of refined carbs, and avoiding natural fats: These might fit the official guidelines of self-appointed experts, but they don't fit the evidence for a healthy diet.

The "fasting lifestyle" I propose is based on ancient wisdom and the Christian calendar, the latest science, the clinical experience of physicians, thousands of case studies, and my own self-experimenting over the last thirty years. The basic idea is simple: we need to become "metabolically flexible," where we can easily run on sugar or fat, and switch from one to the other without feeling like a heroin addict going cold turkey.

To get there, I propose we enter a fat-burning mode called "nutritional ketosis" for at least some amount of time every week. This approach not only mimics the diets and routines of most traditional societies but also allows us to improve on them. That is, we can recover what we've lost as Christians, and as a culture, while taking account of cutting-edge science, and avoiding some of the reasons these traditions disappeared in the first place.

In the following chapters, you'll learn:

- What fasting is
- Why Christians (and others) have fasted throughout history

- When and why most Christians abandoned it
- Why we should still do it
- What spiritual, physical, and mental benefits it offers
- How to alter our diet and lifestyle to make it easier and more sustainable
- How fasting improves our weight and health, where diets fail again and again
- Why we should feast, and how it differs from overeating

Events in the Bible, Christian worship, and history that had seemed opaque and dull will become exciting and transparent. You'll come to see yourself as part of the metabolism of Christ's Body on earth, which is now reaching its two thousandth birthday.

We'll walk through a simple, step-by-step plan for you to adjust your diet and eating. This method will allow you to make fasting permanent, without a lot of fuss, bother, or torture.

We'll explore the scientific evidence, with plenty of references in the notes in case you want to check the facts for yourself. And I won't stand on the sidelines. I've already tried this on myself—going so far as to test blood glucose, cholesterol, triglycerides, hormones, ketones, body fat, and body mass along the way.

The transition plan can (but need not) be fit into one of the penitential seasons of the Christian calendar, such as Advent or Lent. It's forty days plus six little "feast" days on Sundays, so it takes place over forty-six days. Right away, you'll start to acclimate yourself to the pattern you should follow for most of your life: regular eating much of the time, fasting some of the time, and feasting every so often—on different timescales.

Before you start, though, you'll take a few days to prepare. You'll restock your fridge, your pantry, and your mind. There are roadblocks that all of us have to get past before we can really fast. We'll deal with those in the first few chapters, so that you can start the journey with a simple map, a clear mind, and an open road.

Then, in the first week, you'll shift to a "ketogenic" diet of high natural fat, moderate protein, and very low carbs without simple sugars, grains, or starches. This allows your body to shift to a state of "ketosis," in which it draws most of its energy from dietary and body fat. With simple tweaks, you can avoid the nasty "keto flu" that millions of people have suffered during the "induction" phase of the popular Atkins Diet. You'll have a mini-feast on Sunday, when you can let up a bit.

In week two, you'll begin intermittent fasting, which is really just time-restricted eating. Don't worry. We'll start wading in the kiddie pool before paddling out to a deeper 16/8 routine. That is, every day, you'll fast for sixteen hours (including your night's sleep) and eat all your daily calories (mostly fat, protein, and vegetables) during an eight-hour feeding window. And the week will, like every week, end with a Sunday mini-feast.

In week three, you'll work up to a 20/4 routine. That just means you'll eat all your meals within a four-hour window of time during the day. This helps break the habit of eating at fixed times and amplifies the good effects of the ketogenic diet. Then, on Sunday, another mini-feast.

In week four, you'll test out the deep end of the pool for three days—preferably Monday, Wednesday, and Friday. On these days, you'll eat one very large meal over the course of an hour in the evening, but you won't try to restrict net calories.

You'll maintain a time-restricted ketogenic diet on other days. And enjoy a mini-feast on Sunday.

In week five, you'll *mimic* an all-day fast on Monday, Wednesday, and Friday, when you'll consume far fewer calories than you normally do. (Think two avocados with lime juice and salt.) You'll continue with a regular, time-restricted ketogenic diet on the other days. Plus another mini-feast day on Sunday.

In the final week, you'll prepare for and then try a fast of thirty-six to seventy-two hours, and end with a feast. By this time, you should be "fat-adapted" and much more metabolically flexible. You'll have felt the benefits of fasting. Yes, it will still take discipline. But you should find real fasts for three days or more not just tolerable but exhilarating.

This adaptation phase is austere for good reason: if you've spent decades running on sugar, it takes several weeks to reset your metabolism and get you going in a better direction. Don't panic. You won't need to keep such a strict diet afterward. You'll reintroduce whole foods you're used to, though, ideally, you'll leave the standard American diet behind.

Along the way, you'll learn about prayer and fasting traditions that we've lost but should retrieve. We'll explore the different forms of fasting and feasting found in Christian history and discover surprising health benefits to these patterns. We'll learn why Jesus and early Christians fasted, and why our lack of fasting may be holding back a spiritual awakening in our families, churches, and country.

Physically, you'll become insulin sensitive, fat-adapted, and metabolically flexible.

Mentally, you'll enjoy much greater clarity and focus.

Spiritually, you'll be renewed, invigorated, disciplined, and much closer to God.

My goal is to help you enjoy all the fruits of fasting. The fasting lifestyle is about re-integrating the whole person—body, mind, and soul—at a time when we are becoming ever more dis-integrated. Unless you have a medical condition that prevents it, fasting is good for your body, your mind, and your soul. You don't have to take that on faith. You can prove it to yourself in just a few weeks. Want to know how? Keep reading.

CLEARING
THE PATH

1

How and Why Christians Used to Fast

In Scripture and in Church history, Christians fasted for penance. But they also fasted to put their passions and appetites under control, to identify with Christ, to enrich their prayer life, to become holier, and to prepare for spiritual battle.

Strictly speaking, to fast means to freely give up food (and sometimes drink) for some amount of time. People often use the word "fast" to refer to something for which we already have good words: "abstain" and "abstinence." For example, "I am fasting from eating corn chips during Lent." Worse is when the word is used to refer to nonfood items. The Facebook "fast" is a glaring example. This dilutes a perfectly good word. The old *Catholic Encyclopedia*, still a great place to find the traditional Catholic take on all manner of topics, defines fasting this way: "In the strict acceptation of the term, fasting denotes abstinence from food."[1]

That's how it's used in the Bible, too, by the way—going without food for a longer than usual period of time.

That meaning is worth defending against all this loose talk about fasting from Twitter, fasting from soft drinks, fasting from Netflix, et cetera. We need a word to connect what we should be doing to what Jesus did just before the start of his ministry. And to what hundreds of millions of Christians have done for centuries. We have a nice, one-syllable word for that: fast.

Muslims also fast from both food and drink between sunrise and sunset during the month of Ramadan. For many Muslims, this happens during the summer, which means they must go for a longer-than-twelve-hour day without anything. And, since they sleep, they go most of the night without food or drink as well. That includes water! In other words, they must eat and drink only in the very early morning or late evening, just before bed. *For a month.* Compared to that, our little partial fasts on Ash Wednesday and Good Friday are modest indeed.

Still, the Church has long considered it a "fast" when we give up large amounts of food for some period of time, even if we still eat certain foods. We'll call these "fasts" to accommodate this tradition. But we shouldn't forget the primary sense of the word.

Ramadan is a uniquely Muslim fast, anchored in the ninth month of the lunar Muslim calendar. Christians have never given up water during fasts, so far as I know. That makes Ramadan a long, if intermittent, fast. Still, serious fasting isn't a Muslim thing that Christians should avoid. Religions and people feast and fast for all sorts of reasons. Jesus fasted from all food for forty days in the wilderness before he launched his public ministry. At other times, he feasted. So early Christians followed his example, participating in fasts of various lengths and religious feast days.

What Early Christians Did

Why should we care about early Christian practice? Because Christians in the first few centuries were much closer to the life and language of Jesus than we are. They preserved and compiled the New Testament. And for the first three and a half centuries, they lived their lives in a hostile culture that sometimes hunted them down and killed them. So it's easy to see where we've grown lax by comparing what we do with what they did.

And when it comes to fasting, they put us to shame.

The *Didache*, which was written around AD 110—some 250 years before the New Testament was finally canonized—took fasting for granted. It advised Christians to fast and pray for their enemies (you know, the very ones who at the time might be trying to kill them), and to fast for one or two days before baptism.

Although Christians fasted from the beginning, the practice wasn't unique to them. In part, they were following Jewish practice. Even some non-Jewish pagans fasted. But growing tensions between those Gentiles and Jews who followed Christ, and those who did not, led Christians to distinguish their fasts from the surrounding culture. "Let not your fasts be with the hypocrites," the *Didache* advises, "for they fast on Mondays and Thursdays, but do your fast on Wednesdays and Fridays."

Why those days? Because that's when Jesus was betrayed and crucified.

These fasts were nearly universal among Christians, and not just among monks and ascetics.

Fasting for Everyone

Unlike some later Christians, who rejected fasting as a holdover from paganism or Romanism, early Christians didn't think that just because Jews and pagans fasted, they shouldn't. On the contrary, the Church Fathers argued that fasting was intended for the whole human race. They noted that God's *first command* to humanity was to abstain from one kind of food. Adam and Eve could eat the fruit of any tree in the Garden of Eden except for the Tree of Knowledge of Good and Evil. (And they couldn't even manage to do that!) "Fasting is as old as mankind itself," preached St. Basil the Great. "It was given as a law in paradise. The first commandment Adam received was: 'From the tree of the knowledge of good and evil do not eat.' Now this command, 'do not eat,' is the divine law of fasting and temperance."[2] Basil took the command to Adam and Eve to be part of a more general rule, namely, that sometimes we're supposed to refrain from eating.

Basil wasn't alone. All the major Church Fathers—including Justin Martyr, Polycarp, Clement of Alexandria, and Augustine—commended fasting, and saw it as a rule for the whole human race. In a sermon on prayer and fasting, for instance, Augustine—who was not an extreme ascetic—said, "Fasting cleanses the soul, raises the mind, subjects one's flesh to the spirit, renders the heart contrite and humble, scatters the clouds of concupiscence, quenches the fire of lust, and kindles the true light of chastity. Enter again into yourself."[3]

Hard-Core Fasting

St. Anthony (AD 251–356), the father of monasticism, is the superhero of fasting. You might get that sense from the fact that we refer to him as a "Desert Father." That has to mean something hard-core, right? Indeed, St. Anthony said that "true fasting is constant hunger."

Anthony had inherited his parents' wealth around the age of twenty. But instead of resting on his laurels, he took up Jesus's command to the rich man—to sell everything and follow him—by selling everything and moving to a tomb near his home town in Egypt. St. Athanasius tells us that during his time there, Anthony was attacked by both devils and wild animals.

After fifteen years of that, he then retreated to an old fort in the desert. He survived on what little food was tossed over the walls by pilgrims.

After Anthony had spent twenty years as a desert hermit, his followers persuaded him to organize and teach them.

That sabbatical, for which he gained the title "Father of All Monks," lasted for just a few years. He then retreated again to a mountain in the desert. In contrast to his earlier years as a hermit, though, he started receiving visitors. (If you trek to his mountain retreat in Egypt, you can still visit the monastery named after him, Deir Mar Antonios.)

During this last stage of his life, he even traveled twice to Alexandria, the hometown of Athanasius. The first visit was to tend to the Christians there who were suffering persecution under the Roman emperor Diocletian. The second visit came at the invitation of Athanasius, who was busy fighting Arianism—a heresy that rejected the divinity of Christ—which had infected the Church far and wide. After preaching on behalf of Christ's divinity, Anthony returned to his desert retreat.

Despite forgoing baths, wearing a hair shirt, subsisting on little more than bread, salt, water, and sometimes lentils, and fasting every other day, he lived to the ripe old age of 105.[4]

His biography by Athanasius, written shortly after Anthony died, inspired thousands to pursue monasticism. And that became, as *Christianity Today* puts it, "one of the most important institutions in Western history."[5]

For most Christians, Anthony's life is, at best, a curiosity. Mark Galli, an editor of *Christian History* magazine, asks the question that is in the front of your mind: Were the Desert Fathers like Anthony "models or kooks"?[6] Galli thinks they are models. Their stories should be, he argues, a bracing reminder of how little most of us do in trying to follow the Lordship of Christ over our daily lives. Still, the life of the emaciated hermit is not, and cannot be, the calling for every Tom, Dick, and Mary. Most of us are called to marriage and family. Many are called to life in a noisy city. Some are called to homeschool their many kids. The hair-shirt-lentils-and-water routine just won't work.

But—and here's the key point—God did not intend for fasting to be consigned only to the rare monk or hermit. He intended it for everyone. He intends it for you. That's why the Church, in her wisdom, came to include not just feasts, but fasts, in the Christian year.

Lent

Of course, the detailed fasts tied to the Church calendar took a while to develop. Besides the Wednesday and Friday fasts, many Christians began to fast with catechumens (persons receiving training in Christian doctrine and discipline) during the six weeks leading up to their baptism and reception into the Church at Easter. This was perhaps the first instance of truly communal fasts and coincided roughly with Christianity becoming the official religion of the Roman Empire. Christians also came to observe a water-only fast from midnight until the feast of the Mass the next day.

Over the same period, a devotion had grown up around the idea of Jesus's forty hours spent in the tomb. That number forty, of course, reflects a common biblical theme.[7] In the time of Noah, it rained for forty days. Moses fasted for forty days before receiving the Ten Commandments. The Jews wandered in the desert for forty years, while Jesus fasted in the desert for forty days. It's no wonder, then, that by the seventh century, a forty-day Lenten fast starting with Ash Wednesday and ending at Easter had become common throughout Christendom.

By the time of the High Middle Ages, Christians observed not only the long Lenten fast but also the three "Ember Days" that fell at the joints of the four major seasons. (More on those in chapter 24.) St. Thomas Aquinas discusses both in his treatment of fasting in his *Summa Theologiae*.[8]

Things have gotten so soft in recent decades, though, that most Christians have never really seen liturgical fasting in action. To witness it, we have to turn to the Eastern Rite and Eastern Orthodox traditions.

2018 Fasting Calendar

Legend

Abstain from meat, fish, dairy, eggs, wine, olive oil
Abstain from meat, fish, dairy, eggs
Abstain from meat, dairy, eggs
Abstain from meat

January

SUN	MON	TUE	WED	THU	FRI	SAT
	1	2	3	4	5	6
7	8	9	10	11	12	13
14	15	16	17	18	19	20
21	22	23	24	25	26	27
28	29	30	31			

February

SUN	MON	TUE	WED	THU	FRI	SAT
				1	2	3
4	5	6	7	8	9	10
11	12	13	14	15	16	17
18	19	20	21	22	23	24
25	26	27	28			

March

SUN	MON	TUE	WED	THU	FRI	SAT
				1	2	3
4	5	6	7	8	9	10
11	12	13	14	15	16	17
18	19	20	21	22	23	24
25	26	27	28	29	30	31

April

SUN	MON	TUE	WED	THU	FRI	SAT
1	2	3	4	5	6	7
8	9	10	11	12	13	14
15	16	17	18	19	20	21
22	23	24	25	26	27	28
29	30					

May

SUN	MON	TUE	WED	THU	FRI	SAT
		1	2	3	4	5
6	7	8	9	10	11	12
13	14	15	16	17	18	19
20	21	22	23	24	25	26
27	28	29	30	31		

June

SUN	MON	TUE	WED	THU	FRI	SAT
					1	2
3	4	5	6	7	8	9
10	11	12	13	14	15	16
17	18	19	20	21	22	23
24	25	26	27	28	29	30

July

SUN	MON	TUE	WED	THU	FRI	SAT
1	2	3	4	5	6	7
8	9	10	11	12	13	14
15	16	17	18	19	20	21
22	23	24	25	26	27	28
29	30	31				

August

SUN	MON	TUE	WED	THU	FRI	SAT
			1	2	3	4
5	6	7	8	9	10	11
12	13	14	15	16	17	18
19	20	21	22	23	24	25
26	27	28	29	30	31	

September

SUN	MON	TUE	WED	THU	FRI	SAT
						1
2	3	4	5	6	7	8
9	10	11	12	13	14	15
16	17	18	19	20	21	22
23	24	25	26	27	28	29
30						

October

SUN	MON	TUE	WED	THU	FRI	SAT
	1	2	3	4	5	6
7	8	9	10	11	12	13
14	15	16	17	18	19	20
21	22	23	24	25	26	27
28	29	30	31			

November

SUN	MON	TUE	WED	THU	FRI	SAT
				1	2	3
4	5	6	7	8	9	10
11	12	13	14	15	16	17
18	19	20	21	22	23	24
25	26	27	28	29	30	

December

SUN	MON	TUE	WED	THU	FRI	SAT
						1
2	3	4	5	6	7	8
9	10	11	12	13	14	15
16	17	18	19	20	21	22
23	24	25	26	27	28	29
30	31					

What Eastern Christians Do

Step into a traditional Eastern church, and it feels like stepping back in time. These traditions retain much more ancient forms of worship, feasts, and fasts. Check out the 2018 fasting calendar of Eastern Orthodox and Eastern Rite Catholics (eastern traditions that are in communion with the Holy See in Rome) on page 28.

This is a serious regimen. Except when they land on feast days, there are partial fasts every Wednesday and Friday. There are fasts of different kinds for all forty days of Lent (not just mini-fasts on Fridays). And these get more intense during Holy Week. Look at March. All those days marked in light gray are, in effect, raw vegan days.

But wait, there's more!

There's another forty-day fasting period during the weeks before Christmas—though this is not forty consecutive days without food.

And a monthlong fast for the apostles (including especially Peter and Paul) during June.

And fasting periods before a lot of special holidays.

Don't worry. Young children, the ill, and pregnant women are exempt.

This is *not* a starvation diet. Yes, there's plenty of fasting and abstaining from various and sundry foods. But there are also normal days as well as feasts when the faithful eat and drink more than they would on normal days.

When I first saw this calendar, I thought: *I could never pull this off, and, frankly, I don't want to.* I have the same thought when I read about heroic Middle Eastern Christians who choose to go to their deaths rather than renounce their faith in Christ.

You may have the same thoughts.

But here's another thought: What if fasting and spiritual heroism go together? It's hard not to notice that Christians who have survived for centuries in persecution hot spots tend to have the most hard-core fasting calendars. Coptic Christians in Egypt follow a supersize version of the Orthodox calendar. It covers 210 days of the year and is sometimes strictly vegan, or even water-only. The Ethiopian Orthodox have some kind of fast 250 days a year (out of a total of 365)! Some of these are water-only fasts.

What about Chinese Christians? Yep, lots of fasting.[9]

I mention all this not to insist we should do what Ethiopian or Chinese Christians do. My hope is to open up the window of options in your mind. Fasting is not as hard or eccentric as you might think if you've never made it part of your lifestyle. Hundreds of millions of Christians have done it throughout history.

In fact, you've fasted every day of your life. If you've ever finished your last meal at 7:00 p.m., and not eaten again until 7:00 a.m., you've survived a twelve-hour fast! To get serious about fasting, you can start with that first small step, one you've already taken thousands of times.

The word "breakfast" reminds us that fasting was once so common that it found its way into the language used to refer to the first meal of the day. We retain it still as a dead metaphor.

So, why did Christians quit fasting? We'll deal with that question in the next chapter.

2

Why We Quit Fasting

In his book *The Spirituality of Fasting*, Father Charles Murphy describes an encounter he had with St. Pope John Paul II. It was 1980, and they were having dinner at the North American College in Rome. The pope had visited the United States not long before and was puzzled by what he saw. "What happened to fast and abstinence in the Church in the United States?" he asked.[1] The slack fasting of American Catholics stood in stark contrast to the fasting the Holy Father had experienced in his oppressed and densely Catholic Poland.

The problem isn't limited to the US. Christians have been backing away from the rigorous fasts of the early Christians for hundreds of years. For centuries before that, though, Christians on fast days either ate nothing, or at least nothing until sundown, when they might have had a little bread or some vegetables if needed. Over time, full day fasts often weakened into full day abstinences from certain *kinds* of foods, such as meat and dairy. This could be a burden if these were your main sources of sustenance. But it's not much of a mortification if you can eat lobster tail and fish and chips.

The loss of strict fasting really picked up speed over the last few centuries. It is, in part, a casualty of Christian divisions. The great schism of 1054 between East and West marks one big divide. East and West followed nearly identical fasts for centuries after the schism—with some variations owing to their quite different locations. Their practices slowly started to diverge in the fourteenth century.

In the West, the split over the Protestant Reformation, which we can date from 1517, led to an ever more divided Christian world.

Fasting among Protestants has been complicated. Neither Martin Luther nor John Calvin opposed fasting. But both criticized *Catholic* fasts for what they saw as their legalism and works-righteousness. They were convinced that Catholics were trying to earn their salvation by fasting and performing other disciplines. (This was not Church doctrine. Augustine had dispatched Pelagius's view of works-salvation a thousand years before. Still, Calvin and Luther's charge is understandable given the corruption of the times.) Both allowed that fasting, rightly framed, could be good. And many Lutheran and Reformed groups did fast.

The Swiss Protestant Ulrich Zwingli took a much dimmer view of the whole business. While he conceded that a Christian might fast privately to discern God's will, he opposed a requirement of fasting that would impinge on Christian liberty. As a result, he opposed communal fasting such as the Lenten fasts practiced by Catholics as hypocritical and unbiblical. And with that, the liturgical calendar disappeared into the mist. The near-complete ignorance of the Christian year among many evangelicals owes much to Zwingli.

Anglicans and those following John Wesley, in contrast, embraced corporate fasting.[2] Indeed, early Wesleyans made fasting a key part of their spiritual practices, and communal fasts were common in England through the Victorian period. The prominence of these traditions in early colonial America may explain why there were national fast days in the US up until the time of the Civil War.[3]

Since the mid-nineteenth century, though, Protestants have mostly taken Zwingli's lead. Fasting, which was for centuries as much a part of corporate Christian practice as prayer, worship, singing, and the Lord's Supper, became an individual matter—and for many Christians, a nonexistent one. When evangelical Quaker Richard Foster wrote *Celebration of Discipline* in 1988, he said he could not find a single book on fasting written by a Protestant from 1861 until 1954. There were one or two exceptions, but he was right about the trend.[4]

Catholics have retained communal fasting, but these fasts have become ever more watered down and symbolic. Already in 1907, the author of the article on the "black fast" in *Catholic Encyclopedia* could observe, "During the past fifty years, owing to ever changing circumstances of time and place, the Church has gradually relaxed the severity of penitential requirements, so that now little more than a vestige of former rigor obtains."[5]

The encyclopedia's entry on fasting itself, written in 1909, complained, "No student of ecclesiastical discipline can fail to perceive that the obligation of fasting is rarely observed in its integrity nowadays."[6]

That's Arbitrary

So, what caused Catholic fasting to become vestigial? First, the fasts, as we called them, started to seem arbitrary. A straight water fast, which was common in the early Church, is clean and simple. It imitates what Christ did in the desert for forty days. But it's also hard for most people to sustain for long, let alone for days at a time. So, within a few centuries, allowances such as veggies after sundown started to appear. These small snacks, or "collations," then crept earlier and earlier into the day.

At some point, especially in places near the Mediterranean, hungry Christians wondered if shellfish ought to be allowed. After all, John the Baptist, that great abstainer and faster, ate locusts in the desert. And aren't shrimp just sea locusts?[7] By way of this logic, the first sea creatures entered the fasting menu. (For some reason, few pressed for the option of locusts themselves.)

But wait, someone soon thought. *If we can eat shrimp and crab and octopus, what about other seafood? Is it all that different? Didn't Jesus cook and eat fish with Peter and the other apostles on the beach after his resurrection? If it's good enough for Jesus in his glorified body, surely it's good enough for Christians. And by the way, that charbroiled fish filet looks quite tasty.*

You can see where this is going. The complete story is long and winding, and even involves distinctions between more- and less-fatty fish. But the basic trend is simple. It starts with water-only fasts and ends with various and sundry abstinences qualified with ever more quirks and exceptions.

From a historical distance, the whole thing starts to look like a kludge, cobbled together for no clear spiritual benefit. It looks even more arbitrary when a rule that made sense in one time or place gets transplanted to another. Giving up all animal flesh and products, for instance, meant something dramatic to herdsmen and fishermen. It might be a huge sacrifice if you get 80 percent of your calories from lamb or fish, but little if you subsist mainly on sweet potatoes. And if fish is exempt from the category of "meat," and you live next to the ocean, a rule against eating land animals is at most an inconvenience.

One result of these regional differences plus widespread immigration all across the globe? "Meat" in Catholic parlance now refers not to all animal flesh (as non-Catholics might expect), but to flesh from *land* animals such as cows and chickens.[8] Fish isn't "meat."

Another niggle emerged among Eastern and Mediterranean Christians, who struggled over what to do with olive oil. After all, it's sort of like butter. And since butter comes from land animals, is it meat, which means it shouldn't be eaten during stricter fast days? Or should it be allowed on some fast days but not others? In any case, that question never came up for Christians in northern Europe, who knew nothing of olives or their oil.

The second cause of the decline in fasting is surely the long-term effect of local dispensations. Because the Catholic Church has a central authority, exceptions made for one country or region tend to spread. In the US in the nineteenth century, Catholics lived and worked in a largely Protestant country that had ceased to keep strict Lenten fasts. This made it tough for Catholic laborers to keep up. As Orthodox Deacon Joseph Suaiden puts it:

Many low-wage Catholic workers (they got the hardest jobs) were in areas where it was difficult to fast, and they were being converted over to Protestantism because, well, if you're a miner and not a merchant, you don't have much of a luxury to fast. You'll die. So the Popes granted massive dispensations

throughout the Lenten seasons, leaving the fasting season
just a peppering of days varying throughout different regions.
(In South America, however, many of the fasting practices
persisted, even though dispensation filtered its way down.
The easy way always does.)[9]

Notice that the reason for dispensations in the US didn't
hold in South America, where at the time most people were
Catholic. But this is how entropy works in groups. It's much
easier for people to blow off than to take up a discipline.

These days, for Western Catholics, the Code of Canon Law
requires only an hour of "fasting" before communion, no meat
on Fridays during Lent, and two fasting days—Ash Wednesday
and Good Friday—at the beginning and end of Lent. These
aren't day-long, water-only fasts. You can have one regular meal,
with fish (including shellfish of course) plus two snacks that
together don't make up more than one regular meal.[10]

Now picture yourself living in Seattle or Boston or Houston in 2020. You're a faithful Catholic, so you give up bologna
sandwiches on Fridays and Ash Wednesday—which you never
eat anyway. And yet you can still have lobster tail and chocolate
cake—which you love! Or you can have cheese and veggie pizza,
a big bowl of pasta, or a bag of donuts. Or maybe you're a vegan
and don't eat animal products ever. In that case, the sacrificial
logic of the meatless Friday has been lost. Only the bit about eating two smaller meals looks at all like a fast.

Before I studied the history of fasting, I assumed that Vatican II (1962–1965) had weakened most of the rules around fasting. (Catholics often blame Vatican II for anything wayward

they witness in church.) But it's not that simple. Vatican II did make the meatless Friday outside of Lent optional, but the Council fathers still called for Catholics to make a sacrifice every Friday. They had a good reason for this. For most Catholics in the twentieth century, eating fish was just not a sacrifice. It was a mild hassle that looked like a random rule. It had become mere legalism. The bishops hoped to help the faithful recover the earlier idea of penance and sacrifice.[11] Every Friday, in solidarity with Christ, who suffered on Good Friday, we were to give up something meaningful.

But like so many things with the Second Vatican Council, this signal got garbled by the noise of the 1960s. Instead of recovering real sacrifice, most Catholics just started eating meat again on Friday. I didn't learn what the Council really wrote about this until several years after dialing into the issue. Most Catholics still don't understand it.

These days, Catholics, including many orthodox religious orders, tend to abstain rather than fast. Hence, we all "give up" something for Lent. Again, the spirit behind this shift makes some sense: Centuries-old abstinences may seem arbitrary. But that is in large part *because the participants aren't really fasting*. Rather than turning to symbolic gestures to try to make the whole business feel less arbitrary, why don't we recover fasting?

I'm convinced that one reason the Church is so weak is that she has abandoned this ancient spiritual practice. It's hard not to notice that a decline in fasting has tracked closely with a decline in holiness and faithfulness to perennial Christian teaching. I can't prove this decline has been a *cause* of the spiritual weakness, loss of faith, and encroachments of secularism and heresy that now mark the life of the Church. I suspect it's a causal loop: Heresy and spiritual sloth lead to less fasting. Less fasting, in turn, leads to more sloth and heresy.

We can test this. If God means for us to fast, just as he means for us to pray, worship, and obey his commandments, then surely the loss of fasting would leave bad things in its wake. So, for now, let's treat this as a hypothesis: When we don't fast, there's a spiritual cost. And when we do fast sincerely, we should expect a spiritual benefit. We would never doubt such an idea applied to prayer and worship, so why doubt it when it comes to fasting?

Of course, to recover fasting, we have to deal with many impediments that keep us from it. The big one is the fear that it's just too hard. But does it have to be? We take that up in the next chapter.

3

Fasting Doesn't Have to Be So Hard

Many of us never fast because it seems too hard. Unless you're from, say, Crete or Saudi Arabia, and have grown up with a culture of fasting, you probably think, *I can't do it. I need to eat every four hours. If I fast, I'll be so miserable I won't be able to focus on anything else. And then I'll be so hangry I'll become an ax murderer. How can that bring me closer to God?*

These aren't crazy thoughts. We've all missed a meal and felt famished. We search in panic for the fastest relief we can find—Pringles, M&Ms, that dry, half-eaten Krispy Kreme donut in the break room. Just think how bad it would be if we missed two or three meals in a row! First-degree murder starts to seem possible.

Can't Be Normal

What you may not realize is that *this is not normal*. At least it's not normal for humans historically. Our way of eating creates a near-constant need for food, preferably highly processed and carb-rich. Rather than moving from a fasted to a fed state and then back to a fasted state, we stay in the fed state for most of our waking hours. And if we eat as soon as we get up and right before we hit the sack, the fed state even spills into our sleep time.

This wires our bodies to crave constant infusions of sugar— either from foods with lots of natural or added sugar, or from foods loaded with carbs that quickly break down into sugar in the body. Our bodies are designed to be able burn both sugar and fat (from our diet and body stores) for fuel. If you give it carbs, it will burn sugar. If there are no carbs coming in and you use up the stored sugar in your muscles and liver, then the body can do just fine burning fat.

That's how it's worked for most of human history. But most of us now run mostly on sugar all the time. This is not how God designed our bodies to work best. In fact, if our forebearers had needed to follow this eating pattern to survive, we wouldn't be here. The human race would have gone extinct long before we reached our present age of food abundance. Why? Because for most of human history, our ancestors did not have a constant supply of carby foods and refined sugars. They had no refrigeration, for one thing, and couldn't get fruit when it was out of season.

Before the rise of farming, human beings hunted and foraged. That's why we call them hunter-gatherers. Evidence from archaeology and modern hunter-gatherer tribes suggests that ancient humans ate as much wild meat and fish as they could catch. That includes fatty meat and organ meat. Like it or not, we're apex predators, which means we're at the top of the food chain. Our eyes are on the front of our heads—like tigers and wolves— not on the sides of our heads, like deer and bunny rabbits.

Still, we're not strict carnivores. We're omnivores. This is a good thing, since hunting and fishing with primitive tools was hard and often ended in failure. So, while the hunting men sought meat, the gathering women and children collected whatever nuts, vegetables, leaves, seeds, tubers, and fruits they could find.[1] Although some human groups—such as the traditional Maasai—do fine on an all-animal diet, that was not the fare of most ancient humans and is probably not ideal for most people. For one thing, our livers, unlike those of carnivores, can't synthesize vitamin C, so we need to get it from food.[2] And soluble fiber, which we get from plants, helps feed beneficial microbes in our guts.

Outside of the tropics, seasonal changes meant that early hunter-gathers ate fruit only during the spring and summer. Most of that fruit was nothing like the fruit we eat now. Remember, early humans didn't have massive container ships traversing the oceans. Nor did they have refrigerators and freezers in their caves and huts. And the fruits they did have were much tarter ancestors to our apples and berries, since sweet citrus fruit doesn't grow naturally far from the equator. They might have gorged on seasonal raspberries and blueberries in the summer, which allowed them to pack on extra body fat to be used in the lean winter months.

Oh, and the berries weren't as sweet as the tasty treats that we have now. No one ate year-round, deep red strawberries the size of a child's fist—like the ones we can buy at Costco. Think instead of the little wild berries you can find in the forest.

Even in the tropics, no one had the hyper-sweet seedless bananas and oranges we now eat. All of these are the fruits of human ingenuity—pun intended. For some ten thousand years, we've been selecting and hybridizing fruits and grains. Guess what we select them for? Convenience and sweetness.

Until just a few centuries ago, in fact, watermelons had thick skin and were filled with seeds and unpalatable white rinds. The juicy red and seedless core of modern watermelons is the melon's giant placenta, which we have expanded through selective breeding. Wild bananas had big, hard, inconvenient seeds and thick forbidding skin. Wild peaches? A few thousand years ago, they were about the size of cherries, with waxy skin, big pits, and an "earthy" flavor like a lentil.[3]

The transformation of grains has been even more dramatic. We've been cultivating corn for about seven thousand years. It started as a barely edible wild grass. The part we eat now has a volume a thousand times larger than it was nine thousand years ago and has three times as much sugar.[4] "About half of these changes occurred since the 15th century when European settlers started cultivating the crop."[5] It's a similar story with wheat. Indeed, we've gone on a binge hybridizing wheat since the middle of the last century. It's now radically different from the grain man ate for most of history.

We also *refine* grains far more than we used to. A kernel of wheat sprouted or ground by hand with a stone does one thing to the human metabolism. The same kernel pulverized into dust by industrial machinery does quite another. The first breaks down into simple sugar slowly, the latter much more quickly. That's why even your typical loaf of 100 percent whole wheat bread will start to convert to simple sugar as soon as it enters your mouth.

Now, add to this the massive refining and consuming of sugar. In 1700, Westerners ate very little sugar—say, four pounds per year. Even in 1850, we averaged only a few pounds per person per year. Now, each of us, on average, eats well over one hundred pounds of sugar per year.[6] That's 350–500 calories of sugar *per day*, much of it in processed foods that don't even taste sweet to us.[7]

Why does this matter? As we'll see, these trends aren't just bad for us. They make fasting much harder than it should be.

Blessed (and Cursed) Abundance

Paradoxically, most of these problems are the result of what is otherwise a good thing: our bounty. For most of history, people suffered bouts of hunger, and fears of famine and starvation. Compared to us, our ancestors were victims of scarcity. We, in contrast, are victims of abundance. Few of us know the pangs of true hunger. What we feel when it's time for lunch is more habit than hunger. We're like Pavlov's dog who salivated when he heard the bell that he had learned to associate with food. And when we do feel the first effects of hunger after only a few brief hours without food, it's because our bodies are so slow to burn fat. Again, thanks to the carb-intensive, snack-happy SAD.

Does that mean modern farming and technology are bad? Should we abandon our tractors and plows, eat all our food raw, return to caves—or at least to a medieval village—and starve ourselves during the long winter? No. It just means that our abundance has costs as well as benefits. We need to find ways to prune the costs, while reaping the benefits.

If you read deeply in the paleo-diet literature, as I have, you'll be tempted to treat agriculture as if it were a curse, perhaps the result of Adam and Eve's banishment from Eden. This is unbalanced, and unwarranted. We should thank God for agriculture.

Without it, we could never have built cities, civilizations, and culture.

We should also thank God for the advances of the last few centuries, which have allowed billions of God's image-bearers to survive rather than die near birth. Very few people in developed countries starve to death or die from food- and water-borne disease. We should be thankful that Norman Borlaug developed hearty dwarf wheat with stubby stalks that allow the planet to support larger, heartier seeds. Thanks to Borlaug, billions of people in poor countries such as India have grains that prosper in less hospitable climates. Let's celebrate these gains even as we seek to mitigate the health problems these advances have fostered.

Some of the problems are due to simple abundance. Some are due to how we have changed our foods through hundreds and thousands of years of plant breeding. And some are due to how we prepare and eat our food. For instance, there must be some reason that wheat and peanut sensitivity has gone through the roof in recent decades.

There is one other cause, one with the power to amplify the harm of these other factors: bad information. Many of the very experts we trust to tell us how to stay healthy have given us bad advice, especially when it comes to dietary fat. That advice not only harms our health. It makes a fasting lifestyle a pipe dream for most people.

The good news is that more and more experts are coming around.

Since the story is complicated, let's start with a short summary—including what I mentioned briefly above. I'll describe all this in more detail in later chapters.

1. Authorities with white lab coats have told us that dietary fat is bad, and saturated animal fat is superbad. They've promoted industrial seed oils and low-fat diets as alternatives.

2. When the government went on its anti-fat campaign in the 1970s, food companies responded with scads of "low-fat" options. To cover the tasteless cardboard that resulted, they added more sugar. A lot more.

3. We now get most of our calories from carbohydrates.

4. We gorge on highly processed and refined carbohydrates. That includes stuff we think is good for us. Our bodies quickly turn this into sugar.[8]

5. Humans have spent thousands of years selectively breeding fruits, grains, and starches to make them sweeter and easier to eat, cook, and digest. (But note that much of this happened long before the modern obesity and type 2 diabetes epidemic, so at most it is a contributing factor rather than *the* cause.)

6. Unlike our ancestors, we extract sugar from its natural matrix. (That's a problem because sugar's natural matrix helps offset the damage it does to our metabolism.) We drink it, crystalize it, and add it to most of what we eat. It's in 74 percent of the packaged food in the supermarket.[9] Just try to find ketchup with no sugar in it. (It might contain high-fructose corn syrup. That's also sugar.) Most of us are sugar addicts. And our bodies react like an addict's when we go too long without it.

7. We now eat heaps of sugar, over twenty-two teaspoons a day on average—well over a hundred pounds a year! That's over *twenty-five times* more than the average in

1700, ten times more than in 1800, and twice what it was in 1900. Just since 1977, when the government launched its crusade against food fat, Americans have swelled their intake of sugar by 30 percent. We've also swelled our ankles, necks, and bellies. For comparison, you can only keep about one teaspoon of sugar in your bloodstream. It's toxic at much higher levels. So when blood sugar goes up, the pancreas releases insulin, a gatekeeper that sends signals to parts of your body such as your liver and muscles, telling them to store this sugar and get it out of the blood. But your muscles and liver can hold only so much. When they're full, they put up resistance, and the liver starts converting and storing the sugars as fat.

8.   Finally, we eat too often and for too many hours during the day, rather than switching between fed and fasting states.

For those of us who want to fast and eat healthfully, these realities stand like flabby dyspeptic trolls guarding the entrance to the Promised Land.

A Sacrifice, Not Torture

At this point you might think, *Isn't fasting supposed to be hard? It's silly to imagine we can make it a picnic.* This is half right. Fasting is, and is meant to be, a sacrifice. But it's not meant to be an agony. Think of Jesus's words, "My yoke is easy and my burden is light" (Matt. 11:30). We're supposed to bear that yoke and burden daily. Do people attack you for your faith on Twitter? Join the club. Do you have to resist temptation every day? Welcome to the human race. Do you get distracted when you try to pray more than five minutes at a time? Keep trying. These are the burdens we have to bear, because we are weak-willed and fallen. This side of glory, we all have to struggle against weakness and sin. These burdens become lighter as grace remakes us in the likeness of Christ, as we're strengthened by the Holy Spirit, and we are borne along by the prayers of the faithful. The burdens remain, but they do not crush or maim.

But what if, every time you tried to pray, you got a migraine? Or imagine that every time you gave to charity, you suffered severe nausea and vomiting? Or whenever you resisted the desire to insult someone on Twitter, you lost a night's sleep? These reactions would not be a sign that you should just muscle through and try harder. It would be a sign that you're doing something wrong.

Ditto for fasting. If you feel woozy and start seeing stars when you go more than four hours without food, or have obsessive thoughts about Chick-fil-A waffle fries when you miss lunch, or snap at your husband because you missed your 2:00 p.m. Frappuccino, you've got a problem that needs to be fixed.

In these cases, fasting is not the trouble. The trouble is those trolls, those things listed above that make fasting so much harder than it should be.

The Good News

But there's good news. It's not that hard to give the trolls the slip.

Let's take these one or a few at a time, referring to them by their numbers in the list above. First, (1) is false. Natural dietary fat, including animal fat, is your friend. We should reject the recent shift to industrial seed oils and low-fat and high-sugar foods.

Once you make this shift, it takes just a little effort and forethought to overcome (3) through (8) and make fasting (and a little feasting) a permanent part of your lifestyle.

Of course, in earlier centuries, people fasted in part because they had to. They didn't have Grape-Nuts and granola bars and bagels on hand every minute of every day. Nor did they need constant infusions of sugar like we do. They also lived in cultures that had deeply rooted fasting traditions.

This means we have to go out of our way to cultivate a fasting lifestyle.

But before we get to that, we should toss one troll we haven't mentioned off the bridge. He's the one who tells you that fasting is bad for you.

4

Why Fasting Isn't Bad for You

I used to avoid fasting for longer than a night's sleep. Sure, once in a while I'd eat a bit less as a time-honored sacrifice—on Ash Wednesday and Good Friday. And I'd abstain from (land animal) meat on Fridays during Lent. But I was glad I didn't have to endure the fasts of Orthodox Christians—just the vestigial fasts common among Western Catholics.

Grazing

This is not because I'm a spiritual lightweight. Or rather, that's not the only reason. I thought real fasting—freely going without food for many hours or days—undid what I was trying to do with exercise and a healthy diet. Fasting would kick me into "starvation mode," I thought. That is, my metabolism would drop into low gear, and my body would shed muscle and store fat.

As a strength trainer in college, I taught this to fellow students trying to lose weight and get in shape. As a father, I taught this to my daughters. And for decades, I practiced what I preached. Until just a few years ago, here was my daily eating routine:

- A big breakfast right when I got up, with at least three eggs (with one or two egg yolks removed because of fat), half a grapefruit, oatmeal, and sometimes bacon or sausage
- Mid-morning snack—usually a protein shake with skim milk and frozen banana
- Lunch
- Mid-afternoon snack—usually a protein shake or bar
- Dinner
- Mid-evening snack—usually some nuts, berries, or half a grapefruit
- Protein shake right before bed

Rinse and repeat—for decades. I ate like a hobbit who ran the Bag End Planet Fitness.

I got up at roughly 7:00 a.m. and went to sleep about 11:00 p.m. That means I rarely went more than eight or nine hours without eating—most of that while sleeping. I ate over a sixteen-hour time span while awake, and I ate a meal or snack every three or four hours. Because the body takes several hours to process the food we eat, my routine meant that I was almost always in a fed or semi-fed state. My stomach was even processing food deep into the night, because I ate a lot of protein right before bed. That means it took a few hours for my body to process. And sometimes, if I woke up hungry in the middle of the night, I would eat a bowl of instant oatmeal to tide me over until breakfast.

This was the diet of someone committed to health and fitness. I rarely consumed added sugar or sugary drinks. What grains I ate were whole. I exercised frequently—five or six times a week. I didn't smoke, drank alcohol very moderately, and tried to avoid overly processed foods. I didn't carry a lot of extra body fat, especially for someone my age.

I grazed *because* I cared about my health and fitness. Like most people who read fitness magazines and websites, I knew that insulin and blood sugar affect body composition. If you want to hold on to lean tissue while burning and shedding fat, you should keep your blood sugar steady and your insulin low.

Unfortunately, I was also taught that grazing on lots of smallish meals would help with this goal. It would keep my blood sugar steady, with no jarring spikes and drops. This, in turn, would keep my insulin levels low. In addition, I thought grazing gave my muscles a nice stable protein feed, so they wouldn't flee from my body like rats fleeing a sinking ship. I had been told this, after all, by many an expert.

Hence my fear of fasting. I figured it would encourage my body to store fat and shed muscle. And then, when I did eat after a fast, I imagined my insulin going through the roof, and my body storing fat rather than burning it for fuel.

Now, if you're trapped in a box and go two months without food, you *will* lose lean mass—both bone and muscle. But that's not fasting. It's a form of torture prohibited by the Geneva Convention.

More moderately, if you run a calorie deficit every day for months, you will be "hangry," your metabolism will down-shift, and you'll lose muscle. But again, that's not fasting. It's bad dieting.

Fasting Isn't Starving

In the infamous Minnesota Starvation Experiment led by Ancel Keys in 1944–45, subjects were put on low-calorie, carb-heavy diets for twenty-four straight weeks. The goal was to find out how best to treat malnourished Europeans after the end of World War II. Unfortunately, Keys didn't publish the results until 1950[1]—too late to help much in Europe.

Still, it did give us useful knowledge about semi-starvation. The thirty-six subjects—all healthy men—lost 25 percent of their body weight—which was the target for the study. They started out eating a normal 3,200 calories per day for three months to set a baseline. Then, during the six-month test phase, they took in, on average, less than half that amount—1,570 calories per day. The men needed to lose a certain amount of weight every week, and the scientists found that it became harder and harder to get them to lose weight. (Remember this.) As a result, the researchers had to keep reducing the food rations. Some of the subjects ended up with portions of less than a thousand calories a day. For the better part of *six months*.

The men lost a lot of weight. No surprise there—that was the goal of the experiment. But a good chunk of what they lost was lean weight. Their body temperature also dropped by several degrees. They lost interest in sex—a sign of bad health, though perhaps helpful given their circumstances. Worse, they couldn't think straight. They felt cold all the time. Both their strength and their endurance plummeted. Many became depressed and psychotic. And they fixated on food—even in their sleep.[2]

In other words, it was hell on earth.

When we think of fasting, we picture something like this, even if we've never heard of the dreaded Minnesota study. Why? Because we extrapolate from those bad days when we miss a meal, or bad weeks or months when we go on a diet.

The Minnesota Starvation Experiment, though, was not a

test of fasting. It forced men to lose weight by giving them less and less to eat for half a year straight. If a subject stopped losing weight, the scientists would cut his calories some more. Remember, it was designed to test the effects of starvation. It also, unwittingly, tested a low-calorie diet made up mostly of carbs. The poor men subsisted on stuff like bread, macaroni, and potatoes.

In short, the subjects were deprived of food but given just enough of the kind of food that kept them from switching easily to a fat-burning metabolism. The study tells us little or nothing about the effects of fasting—especially fasting done in the context of a quite different way of eating.

Proper Fasting Is Not a "Diet"

Fasting isn't the same as cutting calories, let alone semi-starvation. Eating less and eating nothing, it turns out, have distinct, even opposite, effects on the body—at least in the short term. Fasting is not what most people refer to as a "diet." A diet is when you try to burn more calories than you take in, with the hope of losing weight and keeping it off. You try to "eat less" and "move more," to quote the catchy advice of every nutrition expert ever. It's something you do for a while, and then quit when you reach your target weight, or, more likely, when you give up because someone left a perfectly good cinnamon bun on the kitchen counter.

A proper fast is not like that. When done right, for the right length of time and—as we'll go more deeply into later—when your body is adapted to use fat for energy, none of these bad things need happen.

Your Metabolism Won't Shut Down

Most diets work at first. That's why there are so many of them. When you first cut calories, you lose weight. Ideally, most of the weight you lose is fat rather than muscle or bone. But even then, you soon reach a limit. You find it harder and harder to drop pounds, and the good effects of the diet peter out. That's because diets drag down your metabolism—what is called your resting energy expenditure (REE) or basal metabolic rate (BMR). This is how much energy your body uses doing basic maintenance— breathing, digesting food, circulating blood, keeping warm, and so forth. These functions, far more than short bursts of exercise, dictate how much energy your body uses during the day.

When you limit calories for a prolonged period, your BMR starts to slow down. You also get hungrier and hungrier. Working out more doesn't help much, since that may make you even hungrier. Sheer willpower may keep you going for a while, especially if you believe you won't run out of willpower.[3] But at some point, hunger overtakes almost everyone. Deep hunger is a biological impulse, like the impulse to breathe or sleep. You have short-term control over it—just as you can decide to hold your breath. But given enough time without enough food, the automatic response takes over. If you manage to hold your breath until you pass out, autopilot will kick in and you'll start breathing again—even though you're unconscious.

The impulse to eat is like that, though, unlike the desire to breathe, hunger comes in waves. If you resist the urge to eat, it will subside after a few hours but then return. This is good news for longer fasts—hunger doesn't keep getting more intense throughout the day, or even across a week-long fast. But trying to endure hunger is not a good long-term plan, especially if your body is used to getting a sugar burst every few hours.

Remember those thirty-six men in the Minnesota Starvation Experiment? They grew listless, cold, and obsessed with food. They were able to lose so much weight because they were locked up as part of a controlled experiment. And when their baseline metabolism slowed and they quit losing weight, the scientists monitoring them just slashed their caloric intake even more. Would it surprise you to learn that a few of these otherwise healthy men had to be dropped from the study because they became delusional and did desperate things like eat out of the trash?

That's why, in the normal world outside the lab, dieters regain all their unwanted weight.[4] In fact, even with diet pills and exercise, some 97 percent of dieters return to their blubbery baseline within three years. Most regain the weight within eighteen months. And many end up heavier than they were before, because they've slowed down their previous metabolic rate.[5] The result is not only depressing. It's bad for you.

A normal fast is much different from a diet. When you fast for short periods, your REE (resting energy expenditure) goes *up*, not down! In one study, subjects' REEs went up for three straight days, and only started to slow on the fourth. Even on day four, their metabolic rate was much higher than it was at the start of the fast.[6] They had to fast for five days or more before their metabolism dropped below their starting rate.

This makes sense. The human body is well designed, even this side of the fall. Think of how our ancestors needed to be adapted to the environment for most of our history (not just the last couple of centuries). God's first command to man and

woman was to be fruitful and multiply and fill the earth and subdue it. It would be a bad design if, at the first sign of food shortage, our bodies started to shut down. If all our ancestors had such
metabolisms, we wouldn't be here now. And there would not be
people groups adapted to every climate on earth.

Imagine two Northern European tribes in, say, 8,000 BC
who get all their food by hunting and gathering. It's winter and
they've run out of food. There's very little vegetation around that
they can eat. The men need to be able to hunt before it's too late.

The two tribes are exactly alike, save for one difference. The
men in tribe A get woozy and weak the minute their cave is bare.
The men in tribe B, in contrast, get a nice boost of hormones
that fires them up and makes them want to hunt. This, in turn,
boosts the chances that they will return home with fresh meat.

Which tribe do you think would be more likely to survive the
winter? Now run that scenario for a few thousand winters, and
it's easy to see that a metabolic slowdown at the first sign of hunger would get a tribe weeded out of the gene pool in short order.

In a good design, the body, at least at first, should kick into
a higher gear to help with the search for more food. And when
it's working as it should, that's just what the body does. It se-
cretes energy-boosting hormones like norepinephrine to help
you hunt down and bag fresh game that might require you to
wear it down over long distances.

You Won't Hoard Fat

It's the same story when it comes to fat. A metabolism that shuts
down at the first sign of hunger would be a bad design for a body
with a lot of reserve energy in the form of fat, which describes

pretty much everyone reading this. And guess what? The same hormones that boost energy during a fast also signal the body to draw down the energy reserves on your hips and belly.

You Won't Shed Muscle

Now let's apply the "good design" idea to muscle. To catch an animal—say, a skittish rabbit or gazelle—our ancestors needed clear heads (the brain uses a lot of energy), fast muscles, and energy to fuel them. Let's assume they've eaten well and have plenty of fat and muscle, but then the pantry runs dry.

Does it make sense that their bodies would start burning muscle for fuel right off the bat? Muscle is mostly zero-calorie water plus protein. Your body needs either glucose or ketones (made from fat) for fuel. It would use a good bit of energy just converting muscle protein to fuel. And for the trouble, it would get about 700 calories per pound of muscle burned. Compare that to fat, which packs 3,500 calories per pound. A pound of body weight stored as sugar—glycogen—has only about 400 calories.[7]

So, if fasting mimics the scenario of a hunter-gatherer at the very start of a food shortage, what do you think happens? During a fast, the body *spares* lean mass such as skeletal muscle and instead burns fat.[8] At least that's what it does when it's used to cycling between the feeding and fasting state.

Dr. Jason Fung, the obesity expert who wrote the foreword to this book, puts it well:

> *Let's imagine that we are living in Paleolithic times. During the summer of plenty, we eat lots of food and store some*

of that as fat on our body. Now it is winter, and there is nothing to eat. What do you suppose our body does? Should we start burning our precious muscle while preserving our stored food (fat)? Doesn't that sound pretty idiotic?

It's as if you store firewood for a wood-burning oven. You pack lots of firewood away in your storage unit. In fact, you have so much, it is spilling out all over your house and you don't even have enough room for all the wood you've stored. But when the time comes to start up the oven, you immediately chop up your sofa and throw that into the oven. Pretty stupid right? Why would we assume our body is also so stupid?

The logical thing to do is to start burning the stored wood. In the case of the body, we start to burn the stored food (fat stores) instead of burning precious muscle.[9]

How does this work? During a fast, the pituitary gland boosts human growth hormone (the stuff many bodybuilders inject in their backsides to help them grow abnormal amounts of muscle). This not only helps our body burn fat. It also helps us spare muscle.[10]

That said, if you've been on a constant sugar feed for the last few decades, switching to a fasting lifestyle in one fell swoop can be unpleasant. And that fat-burning system may take a while to come online. That's why it makes sense to prepare your body ahead of time to burn fat. We discuss why in the next chapter.

5

Using Fat for Fuel

If you eat anything like the standard American diet, your body runs mostly on sugar. That means it's really using only one of its two metabolic systems. As a result, your fat-burning system is going to need a jump start. You'll need to make a stark change in your routine, at least for a few weeks. The good news is that it's easier than dieting and, in the long run, it will help rather than hurt you. It won't just help you reduce body fat and improve your health. It will set you up to adopt a powerful spiritual practice that we should never have abandoned.

Your fat-burning mode is called ketosis. That's the metabolic state in which your body converts fats into ketones and uses those, rather than sugar, for energy. (Don't confuse ketosis with *ketoacidosis*, which is a dangerous complication from diabetes in which the body can't produce enough insulin. When this happens, both blood ketones and glucose get extremely high. Unless you're a type 1 diabetic, this isn't something to worry about.)

There are two ways to turn on ketosis:

1. Don't eat anything for three days.

   That's the hard way.

2. Eat a ketogenic diet for several days.

   That's the easy way.

A ketogenic diet is one that is very high in natural fat, very low in carbohydrates, and moderate in protein. And it sticks with carbs that don't fiddle much with the insulin dial.

What does this have to do with fasting? A lot. To make fasting part of your lifestyle, you need to be able to switch between your sugar-burning and fat-burning systems. You need to be *metabolically flexible.* And if you are rarely in ketosis, your fat-burning system will be rusty, sluggish, and in need of a major tune-up.

We'll walk through the details of this in future chapters. For now, here's a simple summary of a very complex story.

You learned in school, as I did, about the three macronutrients—fat, carbohydrates, and protein. Carbs and protein have four calories per gram. Fat has nine calories per gram. That means, we were told, that fat is more than twice as fattening as carbs and protein. Therefore, to avoid eating too many calories, which will make us fat, we should eat a low-fat diet. In essence, avoid fat to shed fat—simple!

Simple but misguided.

This line of reasoning assumes several things. It assumes, first of all, the caloric theory of obesity. That's the idea, which seems self-evident, that you get fat when you take in more calories over time than you expend. The theory focuses less on foods themselves than on foods reduced to their energy content, calories—which are units of energy. So, at least for the purpose of counting calories to lose weight, a hundred calories of cake icing would be the same as a hundred calories of baby spinach or a hundred calories of olive oil.

Now, anybody with even five minutes of knowledge about nutrition will know that you also need to think about things like vitamins and fiber. Cake icing doesn't score well on either of those tallies. But even if we remember those caveats, we're still at risk of going astray if we cling to the calories-consumed, calories-burned mindset when thinking about weight loss and weight gain.

The logic seems like simple math, but neither our bodies nor our foods are simple. Calories don't exist in isolation from actual foods. And not every food does the same thing in your body. The calorie-is-a-calorie claim is true as far as the physics is concerned. Energy is conserved. The first law of thermodynamics holds. But the claim ignores the fact that the body is a highly dynamic and complex system with feedback mechanisms. It responds and adapts to inputs. Calories-in *affect* calories-out. Eat more calories and your metabolism may speed up, causing you to heat up or fidget more. Eat fewer calories and it may slow down, causing you to slow down as well.

And that's just the tip of the iceberg in terms of the feedback mechanisms. Different foods do different things to our bodies. The fixation on calories is due, in large part, to the fact that scientists figured out how to measure calories in food before they understood how hormones regulate everything in our body. The temptation in science is always to treat what can be measured as the only important thing, and to treat the stuff that we can't, or can't yet, measure as if it doesn't matter.

Go back to those hundred calories of cake icing and the hundred calories of spinach. It's not just that the one lacks micronutrients. The food that enters our mouths is mediated by a complex web of hormones, neuronal regulation, and information processing that we're only now starting to grasp. In fact, your body responds to food that you haven't yet put in your mouth, based on your thoughts about it. Remember the salivating chops of Pavlov's dog? The same sort of thing happens to us. A little dose of insulin may enter your blood in anticipation of that big piece of Black Forest cake you're about to eat. Or that you're thinking about eating because I just mentioned it. Sorry.

Your body uses hormones—little messengers for your cells—to control what it does with food. Insulin, a hormone released by your pancreas, is a key player in this story. Insulin works to keep your blood sugar (glucose) levels from getting too high or too low. It's a gatekeeper: it tells your body whether to store extra sugars and fats as body fat, or to burn fat from your diet and from your fat stores for energy.

Carbs raise your blood sugar and so provoke an insulin response. Carb-rich foods include starches, such as corn and potatoes. Some carbs, like sugar and refined grains, *really* spike blood sugar and insulin. When sugar enters the system, the pancreas deploys insulin to send the sugar into your liver and muscles. Leafy green vegetables have carbs, but these plants are mostly water and fiber by weight. Their fiber and other carbs take your body a long time to process, so they don't raise your blood sugar or insulin much. In fact, they probably keep your blood sugar and insulin lower over the long term.[1]

But why do we need insulin to sweep sugar out of our blood?

Because it's dangerous to have too much sugar in your blood-stream for too long. It damages your pancreas and your blood vessels, leading in the end to atherosclerosis. In fact, it harms pretty much every organ in your body.

How much is too much? Well, even though you have about a gallon and a half of blood in your body, you can only safely hold about a *teaspoon* of sugar in your bloodstream. There are about eight teaspoons of sugar in one can of Pepsi! So, insulin helps shuttle excess sugar into your liver and skeletal muscles, where it's stored as glycogen. But these organs fill up quickly. Once that happens, the rest of the sugar gets sent back to the liver, where it is converted to fat and stored elsewhere.

Protein and Insulin

Protein is not a neutral party here. It doesn't really raise blood sugar (glucose), but it does raise insulin—about half as much as carbs do. The effect is muted if the protein comes into your system with plenty of fat and fiber. Protein helps us feel full longer than carbohydrates do. In fact, sugars and processed carbs tend to stimulate our appetites, since they spike blood sugar, which then quickly comes crashing back down.

So, long story short, if you want to keep your insulin low, you should eat *enough* protein to meet your needs, but no more. That will likely be *at least* one-third gram per pound of your ideal body weight. Let's say you're a 140-pound woman, with an ideal body weight of 120. That means you need at least forty grams of protein per day. That's about eight eggs or one and a half cans of tuna. If you're athletic, have a lot of muscle, and work out really hard five or six times a week, you might even need twice or three times that amount. Still, if you want to keep your insulin low, you should not eat more than you need.

Two Metabolic Systems

As mentioned already, our bodies have two separate pathways for converting food to energy. One pathway converts carbs and some protein to glucose—a type of sugar that every cell in your body can use for fuel. The other one converts fats to ketones. But most of us rarely if ever fully use the fat/ketone pathway. We subsist on sugar, which makes fasting hard. That's because our sugar intake has to be recharged every few hours. Our body is like a hybrid car with a backup gas supply that never gets used because the power charger is always nearby. As long as there is electricity left in the battery, it never bothers to make use of the gasoline.

For the most part, these two systems don't run at the same time. As long as you're eating lots of carbs—especially carbs with a high glycemic load, which I'll explain below—your body will just stick with sugar burning and store any extra carbs as fat. In fact, it will even turn protein to sugar rather than bothering to burn fat. Think about that. Your body will *hoard* extra energy from your food as fat on your liver and heart, in between your intestines and pancreas, on your belly, hips, and thighs, and under your chin. But it won't be able to use the fat. No one would do this on purpose. But thanks to decades of bad dietary advice, many of us do exactly this while trying to do the opposite.

Again, a major player here is insulin. Let's assume you're neither diabetic nor pre-diabetic. If your blood sugar goes up, insulin gets the excess out of your blood. If blood sugar is low and you're used to using sugar for fuel, then you'll get the message that it's time to eat. If you can't, or decide not to, eat (as in option one above), you'll deplete the sugar in your liver and muscles. You can store 350–500 grams of sugar (1,400–2,000 calories) in your muscles, and another 100 grams (400 calories worth) in your liver. That's enough to keep an average man going for a day.

Then what happens? If you eat the standard American diet, by now you'll be frantically looking through the cupboard. If it's empty, you'll contemplate the mini Mr. Goodbar with the fuzz and hair on it that you found between the couch cushions. You see, insulin has hormone buddies, such as ghrelin, who by this point will be screaming "Eat something!" to your brain. (It's ghrelin that makes your stomach *growl* with hunger. That little memory aid comes free of charge.) Your liver will then start to convert protein to glucose, through a process called gluconeogenesis—the creation of new glucose.

If you ignore the temptation to refuel the sugar for a while, though, the other metabolic system will start to come online in fits and starts. Your liver will start turning fat from your diet and body stores into ketones, which it can then burn for energy. This is another fuel, a fuel your brain really likes—just waiting to come to life.

But for this to happen in abundance, you need to keep your insulin low for far longer than you would normally tolerate.

If you have been eating heaps of sugars and processed carbs throughout the day over years or decades, your insulin levels never get very low—at least not for long. You'll stay in a fed or semi-fed state. As a result, your cells could very well become *insulin and carb resistant*. They'll put up a fight when insulin comes a' calling, since they can handle only so much sugar. If they didn't do this, your blood sugar would get dangerously low. Instead, your liver, besotted with glucose, will dump some of the excess back into the blood and you'll be back where you started.

So your pancreas has to keep pumping out more and more insulin to clear it from your blood. That spurs your liver to convert the glucose to fat and coerces your fat cells to let in a bit more fat. But these cells aren't infinitely stretchy balloons. At some point, fat cells become insulin resistant. Then the liver has to start storing the extra fat nearby—including around the pancreas, which makes the insulin. This isn't a healthy arrangement long term. In fact, this may be one cause of severe type 2 diabetes, in which the pancreas can't produce enough insulin to clear blood sugar, leading to dangerously high levels of blood sugar. In that case, you might have to start injecting insulin to do the job. And guess what that causes long term? Yep. More body fat.

Think of that elevated insulin as a signal broadcast to every cell in your body: *Burn sugar, convert any extra to fat, then send the fat to storage and keep it safe from everyday use.*[2] Hey, it might not be great wrapped around your intestines and stomach and heart, but it could come in handy during the next famine, right? The body of an obese man with insulin resistance can end up hoarding most of the energy it gets from food as body fat, and still get hungry and weak just a few hours after the man's last meal. He's lugging around a huge cache of food energy, but it's stored in deep freeze, ten stories underground where he can't get to it.

Why Two Systems?

This might look like a screwy system, but it's well designed for what we needed for most of our history. For most of our time on earth, people had to survive lean times and fat times, in winter and in summer. And it was God's plan from the beginning for us to fill the earth. So it should be no surprise that people can live on every continent on earth and get by with diverse diets. (The refined-grain-heavy, three-meals-a-day-plus-snacks routine is a recent experiment.)

Polynesians can do just fine eating fish, coconuts, and breadfruit. The Kitavans on the Trobriand Islands of Papua, New Guinea, eat some fruit, fish, and coconut. But most of their diet is from starchy tubers such as cassava, yams, sweet potato, and taro. The Maasai in Africa stay lean and fit on little more than milk, meat, and blood from their cattle. Until recently, Inuit tribes and some Caucasian scientists who studied them prospered most of the year on little more than blubber and meat, including organ meat, from whales and seals. Recently, some self-testers such as Mikhaila Peterson (daughter of author Jordan Peterson) have found relief from debilitating diseases by switching to an all-meat diet.[3] Clearly the details of human diet and metabolism are more complex than we've been led to believe.

In addition to this diversity of habitats and diets, for many thousands of years people outside the tropics had to endure gaps in their food supply. That means that they had to spend at least some of the time drawing on the body's fat stores. Again, fat is the best way to store food energy, since it's more energy-dense than the other two macronutrients: carbohydrates and proteins.

Every so often, if they were lucky, our ancestors gorged on

sweet berries and an unexpected store of honey. This allowed them to build up body fat they could use when the berries, honey, and other foods became scarce.

Farming brought a steadier supply of grains and other foods. There was honey, for most a rare delicacy. But no one subsisted day-in-day-out on concentrated forms of sugar and loads of pulverized carbohydrates. That's a modern—and for many people, a deadly—invention.

These days rich, middle class, and poor alike (especially the poor) live on a steady drip of sugars and cheap refined carbs that our bodies quickly convert to sugar. As a result, unless you go out of your way to tap your body's fat-burning system, you won't tap it. The fat on your body will be like those worried guests in "Hotel California." They can check out any time they like, but they can never leave. Worse, they won't even be tempted to check out.

Fasting and Feasting

So what does this have to do with fasting? Periodic fasting, with a feast every so often, mimics this older, natural pattern of switching between fed and fasted states. It allows us to use both systems. It harnesses our body's natural design plan far better than the common modern diet. The evidence? When we started eating this way, there was a dramatic spike in what some call "diseases of civilization": obesity, high blood pressure, insulin resistance, inflammation, type 2 diabetes, osteoporosis, various autoimmune disorders, Alzheimer's, and even epithelial cell cancers.[4] These diseases are rare in traditional hunter-gatherer groups, even among their elderly.

Some of these problems may be due to the downside of agriculture, which certainly has plenty of upside. If we look back, though, it isn't so much the diet that started with those distant Bronze Age farmers where we find the worst dietary culprits. With the exception of tooth decay, most of the damage has happened in the last sixty years. It's gotten even worse in the last forty years, since government started to push high-carb, low-fat diets. Type 2 diabetes used to be called "adult onset diabetes," but more and more kids are getting it. Just from 2000 to 2007, diagnoses increased by over 30 percent![5] And some one in three adults is pre-diabetic.[6] Obesity and diabetes now travel together so often that some researchers refer to them as a single syndrome—diabesity.

We're doing something wrong, and the way we eat surely plays a role.

As you might have gathered, though, it's not much fun to go straight from a standard American diet into a water-only fast, especially when you've subsisted on the SAD for decades. That's why we'll follow a much more humane plan in the ensuing chapters—one that will allow you to ease into ketosis before you start fasting. It won't be easy as pie, let alone as easy as *eating* pie. But it also won't be as painful as trying to starve yourself. And by following the plan, you'll be able to give your body the metabolic flexibility our ancestors took for granted.

6

Stumbling into Fasting

The method we'll follow during the forty-six-day plan is based on my own tinkering with several different well-tested fasting programs. It's also based on some fundamental facts about our metabolism that I've learned over the years by accident. The plan is designed to make the transition as smooth and painless as possible.

I didn't have a transition plan to follow when I started fasting. In fact, if I had tried to go straight from the standard American diet to fasting, I probably would have given up. Happily, by the time I pursued fasting I had found my way out of the SAD trap. I didn't escape it all at once. I did so over the course of years of lifestyle changes and serendipitous discoveries.

As I mentioned before, for decades, I avoided dietary fat and grazed throughout the day. I've been picking the fat off of bacon since I was in elementary school and drinking protein shakes right before bed since high school. I trusted what officials told me: dietary fat would make me fat, raise my cholesterol, and lead to high blood pressure, stroke, heart attacks, and other disastrous consequences. Fortunately, by the time I got out of college, I also knew to avoid sugar and processed carbs. Despite the raging debates about the best diet—Atkins, low-carb, high-carb, paleo, Pritikin, Ornish, Protein Lovers, or whatever—everyone agreed on this point.

I paid special attention to the glycemic index (GI), which was invented in 1981 by Thomas Wolever and David Jenkins at the University of Toronto to help diabetics determine how various carbohydrates affect blood sugar. The index labels foods on a scale between 0 and 100. A low-GI food raises blood sugar less, or more slowly, than a high-GI food. Pure glucose is the benchmark, so it has a GI value of 100.

Some of the scores are easy to guess. Jelly beans—little balls of sugar and gelatin—have a GI score of 80. Starchy vegetables, such as corn and potatoes, have a medium-to-high GI value. Non-starchy vegetables are low—around 15 or lower. Fruit juices are much higher than the fruits themselves, since juice is the sugary liquid extracted from the fiber and pulp. We aren't designed to ingest pure sugar every day for years at a time. No one should be surprised that doing so is not healthy.

But the details are much more complex than you might guess. For years, I, along with millions of other people, thought that you could figure out the effects of a carb on blood sugar based on whether it was a simple carb like Coca-Cola or a complex carb like whole wheat. The truth is not so tidy.

For instance, even though wheat is a "complex" carbohydrate with hundreds of sugar molecules strung together, white bread has a GI value of 79. What about those long molecules of wheat? They start to break down into glucose as soon as they enter your mouth. "Healthy" whole wheat bread, which I've been eating since I was a kid, is at 68—not much better than white bread. Table sugar (sucrose) is lower than both at 65!

How can that be? It's because sucrose is made up of one molecule of glucose and one molecule of fructose, the sugar most common in fruit. The body can't convert fructose straight to glucose, so it gets shuttled to the liver for processing. As a result, it has only a slight immediate effect on blood sugar. (It does have other bad downstream effects, such as insulin resistance and fatty liver.) That means that only half of every teaspoon of table sugar spikes your blood sugar, which in turn raises insulin.

Corn flakes and other processed cereals can be as high as 84 on the index, even though they are made from "heart healthy" grains. (That's why I ate oatmeal for decades. It doesn't spike blood sugar as quickly as processed cereals.) How food is processed can make a big difference in its glycemic effect. Unprocessed sprouted and whole wheat berries score lower on the index than finely milled flour. Alas, the latter is the form of wheat most of us consume without thinking about it.

The glycemic index has helped millions of diabetics control their blood sugar without recourse to insulin. But it's never been shown to be all that useful for losing weight, because it fails to capture a lot of nuances. The same food, for instance, can have a different glycemic effect depending upon how ripe it is. Even its temperature and how it's cooked can make a big difference. Boiled yams are lower on the scale than roasted yams. Cold rice is lower on the index than warm rice.

Moreover, the index doesn't capture the fact that glycemic responses vary from person to person. Some people are quite sensitive to rice, for instance, while others are not.

The biggest deficiency with the glycemic index is that it fails to account for typical portion sizes of foods. It compares a fixed amount of one hundred grams of carbohydrates of all the various foods. Not a one-hundred-gram serving, but one hundred grams of net carbs of each different food. To get that many carbs of spinach, however, you'd need to eat over six gallons of raw or three gallons of cooked spinach! That's impossible to do in one sitting. Even a tenth that much spinach would be a stomach-stretching salad. In contrast, you could down just a little more than a pint-size bottle of Coke to get one hundred carbs. And guess which option will leave you feeling full longer!

To fix this flaw in the index, scientists developed the concept of a glycemic load, which considers not just the sugar-raising properties of different carbs, but the amount of carbs in a normal serving. To find the glycemic load of a food, you multiply its score on the glycemic index by the number of grams in a portion and then divide by one hundred.

Don't worry about memorizing that. Just remember that some high-GI foods have a low glycemic load. Watermelon, for instance, is a scary 72 on the glycemic index, but by weight it's mostly water and soluble fiber. So its glycemic load is very low, meaning it will have a much lower glycemic effect than you would expect if you used just the index to decide what to eat.[1]

The glycemic load measure is an advance, then, on the bare bones glycemic index, and it has a place. It's limited though. It focuses on blood sugar—important for diabetics—but it doesn't measure insulin, the more likely culprit in obesity and other metabolic diseases. Yes, blood sugar does raise insulin, so the glycemic effect is a major contributor. But blood sugar is not the only thing that raises insulin. Protein can, too, to a lesser degree.

There are a bunch of other fussy details we don't need to get into here. What we really want to know is how insulin levels and insulin resistance are affected by what, when, and how often we eat. The impact of various kinds of carbs on blood sugar is only part of that picture.

I didn't fully grasp all these nuances until about seven years ago. For decades, I was armed with knowledge of the glycemic effect of carbs. So I stayed away from sweets and drank a lot of Diet Coke and Diet A&W Root Beer. I doubt that I've had an entire serving of a regular soft drink in twenty years. And informed by the official low-fat wisdom, I ate a lot of low- and zero-fat food: I Can't Believe It's Not Butter! spray; translucent skim milk with its trademark gray-blue pallor; and dry, soul-depleting skinless chicken breasts.

Yeah, dark days for this first-worlder. But brighter days were ahead.

Big Fat Surprise

It was around 2009 when I started to doubt the official story about dietary fat. I had known since the 1990s that the low-carb "Atkins" diet could help people lose weight. I watched a colleague lose thirty pounds over the course of a few months eating mostly cheese and steak. There were a few years in the late 1990s when I seemed to meet someone every day who had tried the diet with great success—at least in the short run.

The theory made some sense: If you cut out sugars and other carbs and eat a lot of protein and fat, your body will have to burn fat. Simple enough. (Only later did I learn that protein also affects insulin.) Still, I felt sure it was not a *healthy* way to lose weight—so sure that I didn't study the issue. Why bother? Wasn't it obvious that fat—with its nine calories per gram—made you fat? And didn't every nutrition headline announce that fat led to all sorts of health problems?

Those headlines, however, might have been what planted the first seeds of suspicion. If you have read diet advice headlines for the last thirty years, you may have noticed how the conventional wisdom on fats kept changing: One day we were told that eggs are bad for you since they're filled with cholesterol. The next day we were told eggs are good for you. For years we were told to dump butter and eat margarine and industrial seed oils instead. Then we found out that the trans fats in margarine and Crisco are much worse than the butter and lard they were supposed to replace. For years, we were told to watch total cholesterol. And then, every year or two, some new detail would emerge to complicate the official story. In the 1970s, no one would have imagined that Americans would, decades later, be talking about "good" and "bad" cholesterol. Or that later Americans would believe, at the same time, that saturated fat is bad for you, but that avocados (which contain saturated fat) are good for you.

Enough of these contradictions pile up, and you start to doubt the received wisdom. When that happens to me, I tend to study the issue. In this case, I began to research the fat controversy. The books that did the most to change my mind were *Why We Get Fat* and *Good Calories, Bad Calories* by *Science* magazine writer Gary Taubes, and *The Big Fat Surprise* by Nina Teicholz.[2] Honorable mention goes to *Death by Food Pyramid* by nutrition writer Denise Minger.[3]

These books demolish the so-called diet-heart hypothesis, first proposed by Ancel Keys in the 1950s. It is from Keys that we got this argument:

1. Saturated fat raises total cholesterol.
2. High total cholesterol causes heart disease.
3. Therefore, to prevent heart disease, we should lower saturated fat in our diets.

It turns out that there was only decent evidence for (1)— and we now know that total cholesterol doesn't tell us much, if anything, about long-term health. From the beginning, (2) and (3) have been assumptions in search of evidence; evidence that never turned up, even after multi-year, multi-million-dollar double-blind clinical studies. What little evidence there was rested on observational studies where subjects had to try to re-member what they'd eaten over the last several months to years. National dietary advice should *never* have rested on such flimsy foundations. In the years since Americans started following gov-ernment advice and reducing their intake of saturated fats and loading up on the grainy-base food pyramid, diabetes, obesity, and heart disease have shot way up.

A 2017 *Lancet* study revealed the toll a grain-heavy diet has taken on health around the world. Cardiologist Bret Scher explains:

> *The largest-ever analysis of diet, which included 135,000 people in 18 countries, revealed that people who consumed high-carb diets were 28 percent more likely to die during the study than people with lower carbohydrate intake. By contrast,*

those who consumed the highest amounts of saturated fats had the lowest rates of stroke.[4]

When I first read *Why We Get Fat* in the summer of 2013, I began to rethink everything I thought I knew about fat, though the process would take me a couple of years to work through. It's hard to shed biases in one fell swoop. Within a few months, though, I wanted more than mere book learning. So I decided to test Taubes's argument that sugar and carbs, not dietary fat, are the real nemesis of good dietary health. I have no power to control anyone else's diet, so for the subject of the test, I chose myself.

My family and I were living for the summer on Vashon Island near Seattle, just before we moved to Washington, DC. We were preparing most of our meals. I decided to cut carbs and boost the fat in my diet, but not try to cut calories. What I found was that if I kept carbs below 100 grams a day (which is low, but not low low), and avoided sugar, I could eat as much as I wanted, and my body weight stayed the same. The switch caused no detectable harm to my health. I felt fine. My blood pressure and cholesterol stayed normal. If anything, I was stronger and more energetic than I had been before. I wasn't being careful with types of fat at that point. I just boosted fat and dropped the carbs and sugar. Not that complex.

Yes, I know this is an anecdotal n=1 experiment. It isn't scientific proof. I'm not saying you would have exactly the same results. But it was more than enough evidence for me to pursue the question with vigor. What I found was this: None of the efforts by the conventional-wisdom empire to refute Taubes, Teicholz, and others have been at all persuasive.[5] They have merely confirmed that the low-fat high-carb diet advice of the last half century has had little to do with solid science. I had discovered the joys—and science—of fat, and there was no looking back.

It would be another four years before I first glimpsed the physical effects—and the joy—of fasting. By accident.

Finding Fasting

For decades I've had three chronic health problems. One is allergies and a tendency to get colds and sinus infections. (I've had sinus surgery twice so far.)

The second—chronic and acute migraine headaches—I've had since junior high. Fortunately, a combination of drugs and exercise has kept them at bay—though not without side effects.

The third problem, which started in about the sixth grade, is with my esophagus. If I'm not really careful to chew my food and take tiny bites, food gets stuck about midway between my mouth and stomach. Sometimes I can force it down with big gulps of water and willpower. Other times, the food won't budge, and the water comes back up whence it came. This is awkward if I'm at a dinner party.

As a kid, my parents chalked it up to "nerves," as did nurses when I would tell them I couldn't swallow big horse pills—pills that promptly came back up when they told me just to chase them down with a gulp of water.

In grad school, I finally had a heretical thought: *Maybe this is a real medical problem.* So I went to a gastroenterologist. He x-rayed my esophagus and told me I had a severe stricture in the very spot where food always got stuck.

This was good news. It wasn't all in my head! It was a plumbing problem, which, I learned, was easy to fix. Putting me under light anesthesia, the doctor sent a tube with a balloon on the end down my throat. Once it was in place, he then expanded the balloon to stretch my esophagus and relieve the problem. Alas, the effect was temporary, so I was obliged to have this done several times over the years to keep the problem under control. There were other tests to try to find the cause. The usual suspects—such as acid reflux—were ruled out. So I just treated it as a cross to bear.

Then, when my family and I lived in Seattle, I made an appointment with a young new gastroenterologist at the University of Washington health center. He listened as I described the problem, and then he said, "I bet you have eosinophilic esophagitis" (EoE). This was how I learned that the malady *had a name*. A biopsy confirmed the diagnosis. EoE is a disease in which certain white blood cells (eosinophils) fill the wall of the esophagus, causing it to stiffen and swell. This reaction, in turn, makes it hard to swallow.

Getting the diagnosis was good news. The bad news? No one knew what caused EoE. There was an oral steroid spray I could use to reduce symptoms, but it caused thrush, a painful yeast infection in the throat.

A few years passed. My family and I moved to Washington, DC. I had to find another doctor to get my eating tube stretched. Since I would be under anesthesia, I asked the doctor if he could do a twofer: an endoscopy and the dreaded colonoscopy, which I'd never had done. He agreed, but it meant that I'd need to fast ahead of time for about thirty-six hours. I agreed.

I asked him if anything was known about the cause of EoE,

since it had been several years since my last endoscopy. "Have you ever tried the six-food elimination diet?" "No, I've never heard of it," I told him, thinking to myself, *There's no way we're going to fix this with a diet.* He then explained that recent studies on EoE had found that in most cases the condition was the result of food intolerances or sensitivities that often didn't show up in allergy tests.

I was skeptical. How could I have an intolerance to a food I ate every day, and not even know it? I already avoided the foods I was allergic to—lentils and a few nuts like pistachios and cashews. Still, I decided to try the elimination diet after the gastro double-whammy was over.

The night before the procedures, I had already gone twenty-four hours without eating. I decided to work out, assuming I would be weak as a kitten. Instead, I felt weirdly strong and energetic. My mind was also strangely lucid, as if I'd taken a brain-boosting pill. I knew something unusual was happening.

The next morning I had the procedures as scheduled. No colon problems—yay!—but the endoscopy confirmed that I had EoE. Later that day, I started the six-food elimination diet. It required me to avoid the six most likely culprits—for three months. It was November, which meant that over Thanksgiving, Christmas, and New Year's I would not be eating eggs, dairy, wheat, soy, nuts, or seafood. It wasn't easy. But I was determined to do it right.

I dimly hoped I would start to notice something after a few weeks. Instead, my swallowing started to improve . . . in three days. For over three decades, I had been three days away from a cure, and didn't know it.

Within three weeks the problem was almost gone. I was so

used to forcing every bite down with a gulp of water that I had to train myself not to do that.

At the end of the three months, I started to reintroduce foods, one at a time.

I reintroduced dairy first, which I was pretty confident wasn't the problem since my ethnic heritage is entirely northern European. (Europeans are much more likely to tolerate dairy than Asians are.) I started with a dash of heavy cream in my morning coffee. No problem. That evening, figuring the coast was clear, I ate half a dozen cheese sticks. Bad idea. Food was sticking in my throat the next day. I got severe stomach cramps and felt sick for a couple of days afterward. A couple of other self-tests confirmed it: no dairy for me.

This was when I learned that if you eliminate a food that's causing trouble, once you re-introduce it the problem can be pretty obvious.

Over the next few months, I figured out what I could and could not eat. I suspected eggs might be a problem, because I'd had an allergy to them as a kid, which I'd outgrown. Sure enough, if I ate eggs, my throat tightened up.

Long story short: the biggest offenders, starting with the worst, were dairy, eggs, wheat, walnuts, and (for some reason) farm-raised salmon from Costco.

Cutting dairy and eggs from my diet meant that I had to give up half of what I was used to eating. No more omelets or feta cheese or whey protein shakes, or even an occasional pizza. But the trade-off has been worth it. As long as I don't slip up at a reception and eat the mystery hors d'oeuvres, I'm now free of a frustrating problem I've had most of my life. I also suspect that getting rid of these food irritants has helped in other ways. For instance, I no longer have migraine headaches, and my chronically sore back has gotten much better.

Aside from the sheer inconvenience of giving up eggs, dairy, wheat, and everything containing these foods, the discovery of food sensitivities was disquieting. If I could cluelessly eat something for decades that caused such severe symptoms, what other stupid things was I doing? Should I try to eliminate other foods? Should I worry about pesticide residue on fruits and vegetables? What about all the electromagnetic signals from cell phones and Wi-Fi routers?

No one can investigate every possible problem. Besides, an elimination diet has its own risks. It might even cause you to become sensitive to a food you had no problem with before.[6]

Still, the experience compelled me to do research. I started reading everything I could find about food intolerances and sensitivities (as opposed to simple allergies). I became acutely aware of how an unassuming food choice could, over time, devastate one's health. And that's when I stumbled upon the growing literature, and testimonies, about the wonders of *fasting*. They caught my eye because I remembered the moment of clarity and energy I had had during the fast just before my medical tests.

I'm sure that sequence of events was key. If I hadn't had that experience—a forced fast while eating a low-carb diet—and hadn't already known about the glycemic effect of carbs, the effects of carbs on insulin and blood sugar, and the safety of natural dietary fat, I would have been skeptical about the case for fasting. But as it was, I realized that this might be a missing piece to the puzzle. Fasting and the fat-burning state known as ketosis were often treated separately. Now I began to see how they fit together.

Fasting?

Soon I was experimenting with time-restricted eating, intermittent fasting, the fasting-mimicking diet, alternate-day fasting, one-meal-a-day fasting, and longer water-only fasts. It wasn't long before I wondered why Christians had abandoned this practice.

At first, it felt like I was stumbling upon one thing after another. Looking back, though, it seems providential. I'd hate for others not to find what I found, just because they have not traversed the same twists and turns that slowly got me to the top of the mountain. So that's the purpose of the plan that follows: it will allow you to benefit from what I've learned, but to do it in forty-six days rather than twenty-five years. The result, I hope, will be that you are inspired and assisted to shift to a healthy, permanent, eat-fast-feast lifestyle.

7

Prepping for Success

Have you ever counted the days from Ash Wednesday to Holy Saturday? If you have, you found there are actually forty-six days—Lent's forty *fast* days plus six Sunday feast days. Those feast days aren't cheat days added in the sixties. They have punctuated Lent for centuries. And it all culminates with Easter Sunday, the great feast of the resurrection.

Perhaps it's just a coincidence—or perhaps not—that for most people who aren't adapted to burning fat for fuel, it takes about this much time—five to six weeks—to get things humming.

Our transition phase follows this pattern. It's a forty-day plan, with six mini-feast days on Sundays. You can start it at any time of the year, but it fits nicely in the season of Lent.

In theory, you could stretch out the plan over three months, spending two weeks on every week of our plan. But stretching it that long could make it easy to get distracted or to become discouraged by how distant the goal remains.

Alternately, you could compress it into just three weeks. If you've never really fasted, though, I wouldn't recommend that. Diving headlong into ice-cold water is not the best way to learn how to swim. In fact, for a few days before you start, you'll need to prepare.

Then, during your first full week, you will slowly shift from a sugar-burning to a fat-burning metabolism, called ketosis. That's the gateway to successful fasting. If you've tried and failed to fast in the past, it's probably because you were working at cross purposes with your metabolism. Fasting takes discipline and practice. But it's not supposed to be torture.

Once you're in ketosis, you will start to limit the amount of time during the day when you eat. Within three weeks, you'll spend most of your day in a fasted rather than a fed state. For the first four weeks, though, you won't try to reduce the net number of calories you take in over the week. Only in week five will you start to do that. And by the end of the program, you'll be far more flexible in moving to and fro between your fat-burning and your sugar-burning systems.

Fasting, like prayer or riding a bicycle, is a skill. It takes practice, and you can expect to take a tumble and skin your knee a few times. For it to become a genuine virtue, though—for it to become a fixed part of who you are—it first must become a habit. If you stick with the plan, by the end, you should have all the tools you need to make fasting, including multi-day fasts, a part of your routine for the rest of your life. And that life will be much richer, and likely longer, than if you had never taken up an eat-fast-feast pattern in the first place.

Clean Out the Pantry

One of the main hurdles to success early on will be in your fridge and pantry, and perhaps even other places in your house.

There are some treats that tempt you above all others. They call out to you if they're anywhere nearby. Is it Peanut Butter Crunch cereal? Klondike Bars? Cheese-Its? Lay's potato chips? That jar of Jelly Bellys on the coffee table? Maybe you struggle with just a few foods. Or perhaps you love pretty much all the processed delights that occupy the broad middle of every grocery store (away from the outside walls). In that case, you have some work to do. Better get a pen and paper, browse your home for the many dietary stumbling blocks, and write down all their names.

For me, it's tortilla chips. If there is an open bag of corn chips within walking distance, I just can't leave them in peace. I must eat them as soon as possible. I have a whole arsenal of mental justifications for doing this. I especially like the thin, greasy chips we get from a local grocery store, and the Kirkland brand of stone-ground organic tortilla chips from Costco. The easiest way for me to avoid eating tortilla chips is—wait for it—not to have them in the house.

The point is so obvious that I shouldn't have to write about it. But there it is. We're creatures of habit who are easily tempted. If we see something we really like in a moment of weakness, we tend to target it, like Homer Simpson going after the last donut in the church basement.

So if you want to shift to a fasting lifestyle, do whatever you can ahead of time to avoid culinary temptation. Set up trip wires between you and failure. Take countermeasures so that, when you start to cave, you will need just a little willpower to resist. Don't make it easy to fail. Give away or throw away the sugary drinks and treats, and the highly processed treats that you can eat right out of the bag or the box. If you have a family and can't control what's in the house, push to get the off-limits foods as far out of sight and reach as possible. Put notes on the most tempting no-no foods if that's what it takes. Then focus on what you can eat.

Commit yourself for the next few weeks to eating whole food that still looks more or less the same as it looks in nature. Next, stock up your fridge and pantry with the many whole foods that will make up the lion's share of your diet. I'll explain the details in the next chapter. But the general rule for this program is simple: Especially at the beginning, you'll eat plenty of natural fat and moderate amounts of protein, and you'll avoid sugar, starches, and refined carbohydrates. You'll get most of your carbohydrates from vegetables, especially green vegetables that grow above ground. They will take up room on your kitchen counter, on your plate, and in your refrigerator.

You will slow down and actually taste these foods as you eat them. Before long, things that didn't taste sweet enough will start to taste plenty sweet. Your mouth's ability to detect and enjoy subtly sweet tastes will ramp up. (A friend who cut back on sugar said that even butter started to taste subtly sweet to her, and butter has exactly zero sugar!) At the same time, you'll rediscover the pleasure of foods that are tasty without sugar, foods that appeal to other parts of the palate. There are a lot of great foods and recipes that have been crowded out by the SAD's phalanx of added sugars and quick-and-easy carbs. You'll discover or rediscover many of these healthier tasty dishes in the days and weeks to come.

Aren't sure what to buy? No problem. Below is a starter grocery list. You don't have to buy all of the items right off the bat. And there may be one or two that you can banish into the outer darkness. For instance, there is a chemical in Brussels sprouts that only some people can taste, and if they can taste it, these veggies taste awful. If you're such a person, you don't need to force them down. Ditto if you have an allergy to this or that item. There are plenty of good alternatives. The key is to greatly expand the volume and variety of healthy items from these groups, and to do so before you start on your first week.

Groceries

Natural Fats
  Olive oil
  Coconut oil
  Butter
  Ghee (clarified butter)
  Lard
  Tallow
  Avocado oil
  Peanut oil
  Heavy cream

Meat and Protein
  Eggs
  Salmon
  Sardines
  Chicken (including the dark meat and skin)
  Pork (including fatty portions)
  Sausage (make sure it's low-sugar)
  Ground beef (no leaner than 85 percent)
  Steak

Vegetables

Spinach

Bok choy

Broccoli

Asparagus

Lettuce

Kale

Celery

Brussels sprouts

Zucchini

Leeks

Peppers

Onions

Watercress

Cauliflower

Green beans

Snow peas

Seaweed

Artichokes

Cucumbers

Tomatoes

Avocados

Olives

Okay, the last four are technically fruits (the seeds give them away), but they're good to have.

Resist the temptation to get the leanest meats. You will be increasing your intake of natural fats, while moderating your protein. If you eat a lot of grilled ground turkey breast, skinless chicken breasts, mahi-mahi, and egg-white omelets, you could very well end up with too much protein and not enough fat. I know this contradicts everything you thought you knew about a healthy diet. Just roll with it for now.

Nuts and Seeds

Macadamia nuts

Pecans

Almonds

Walnuts

Brazil nuts

Hazelnuts

Pistachios

Sunflower seeds

Pumpkin seeds

Secret Weapons

Dark chocolate (85 percent or higher)

Konjac-root noodles

Frozen "riced" cauliflower

Coffee

Tea (black, green, herbal)

Wait, Where's the Fruit?

This isn't a complete list of your diet for the next few weeks, but you might wonder where the fruit is. Haven't we been told to eat lots of fruits and vegetables, since they're good for us? Yes, but there's actually no good reason to treat these foods under one heading. Most fruits are high in sugar, whereas most vegetables are not. So eating much fruit during your transition will keep you from getting into ketosis. Remember, we've bred fruits to be much sweeter than they used to be in nature. There are some fruits that don't have this problem, ones that may be a part of your healthy eating patterns long term, such as grapefruit, cherries, and blueberries. But even these fruits are sugary carbs. Remember, we're breaking your body of the carb/sugar-for-the-bloodstream-all-the-time habit. That involves some intense, even shocking experiences. You'll get the fiber, vitamins, and other micronutrients you might have been getting from your fruit intake from other whole foods— the vegetables and some nuts that will make up a much larger slice of your daily food intake during the transition.

Natural + Supernatural

Last but not least is something you can't buy at the grocery store—prayer. Take time to pray for guidance and willpower. Unless you are exempt for age or health reasons, then you're supposed to fast. Given that fact, is there any doubt that the Holy Spirit will help you do it if you ask him to? Also, pray about matters unrelated to food. Praise God for his wonderful attributes. Thank him for the many blessings in your life. Practice intercessory prayer for others. This will help remind us that "man does not live by bread alone." Food is a good and essential part of our lives, but it is not the most important thing. A well-rounded prayer life helps us remember this.

WEEK ONE

8

Hello Fat, Goodbye Carbs

After taking a few days to prepare your mind and your house, you can now start to eat in a way that will deplete the stored sugar (glycogen) in your muscles and liver. In your first week, you need to drop sugar and eat fewer than fifty grams of carbohydrates a day (not counting fiber), mostly from leafy green vegetables. To make up for the lost carbs, you're going to eat more fat. In fact, you'll get about 80 percent of your calories from fat.

You might fear that this will cause your blood sugar to plummet. Don't worry. Unless you have diabetes or are seriously prediabetic, your body has a toolkit of hormones to keep your blood sugar within a narrow range. Though it varies between the fed and fasted state, your blood sugar should stay in the normal zone.

Wait, you may be thinking. *Doesn't the brain need glucose to survive?* It does. But your brain can use another fuel—ketones—when sugar is low. It will still need some glucose, even when you're fasting, but it doesn't need any sugar from your diet to get glucose. If there is no sugar coming in, your body will start using extra proteins to produce it in a process called gluconeogenesis (literally: creation of new glucose). It can even get glycerol from fat molecules and use that to make glucose. You can't live long without fat and protein. But there is no essential carbohydrate. You could live for decades without carbs. I'm not saying you should do that, just that you could. So don't worry that you're trying something crazy here.

Of course, your body will still *want* carbs—at first. Old habits die hard, especially ones forged over decades. You may even have an addiction to wheat, which is more common than you might think.[1] Soon, though, if you keep your carb intake really low, your body will get the hint. Your liver will start converting your dietary fat into ketones—acetoacetate, beta-hydroxybutyrate, and a by-product called acetone. Your body will use the first two for fuel.

There will be bumps and false starts as the new system comes online and your body gets used to producing and running on this other source of energy. You might feel odd for a few days, and your gastrointestinal system may need some time to adjust. But if you stick with the plan, your body will switch into fat-burning mode. The process takes about seventy-two hours to start up—three days. If you work out hard, you might even deplete your glycogen stores and start producing a lot of ketones in as little as forty-eight hours.

Why Do I Need to Eat Fat?

But if severe carb restriction (below fifty grams a day) forces your body to turn fats into ketones, why eat so much fat? Why not just eat protein and wait for your body to burn body fat? If you're already insulin sensitive and metabolically flexible (more on that later), that strategy might be okay for a short time. But, remember, protein also raises insulin. Your body can turn protein into sugar, which it will want to do if you're not fat-adapted. So eating nothing but protein is not a good way to turn on the fat-burning system, especially not when you're first trying to make the switch.

Even after the switch, it takes the body a few weeks to learn to use ketones efficiently. You don't want to interfere with that process. If your body is not used to drawing on fat stores for energy, dropping most of the carbs from your diet is a stressor by itself. Cutting out dietary fat at the same time is too much like a straight-up fast. (If you cut out protein, too, then it *is* a fast.) Remember, the goal is to make fasting part of your everyday life, not to try it once, hate it, and never try it again. You need to break old habits. Feeling famished right off the bat is not a good way to do that. Trust me. It's much better to eat extra dietary fat while your body is adjusting to its alternate fuel source.

For your first week, eat as often as you normally do. Don't overeat, but don't try to cut back either. If you're hungry, eat food. If you're thirsty, drink water. Even when you aren't thirsty, drink water. One of the first things your body will do when you cut carbs is shed a lot of water. So you'll need to compensate for this.

The basic rule for this week is simple: Natural fat is your friend. Sugar, most carbs such as grains, and starches are your enemies. For the next few weeks, you will abstain from them— with mini-exceptions on Sundays, your feast days. Think olive and coconut oil, meat, eggs, hard cheese, nuts, spinach, asparagus, and salad galore. Forget Coca-Cola, pasta, bread, potatoes, cereal, donuts, candy bars, all fruit juice, and most fruits.

Get most of your calories (at least 75 percent) from natural fat found in oils, meat, eggs, and nuts. Get as much protein as you need, but no more than 20 percent of total calories should be protein. Eggs and every form of meat contain protein. Get only a tiny amount from carbs (about 5 percent of total calories), mostly from vegetables. For most of us this means keeping your total *net* carbs under fifty grams a day. Others will need to drop net carbs even more. (See appendix 3 for more information.)

Here's what net carbs means. Strictly speaking, fiber is a carbohydrate, but it has a negligible effect on blood sugar and, by lowering the glycemic effect of other foods you eat at the same time, probably makes you more insulin sensitive long-term. Fiber also blocks the bad effects of other carbs. So, for now, you can subtract the fiber from total carbs. Let's say you eat carbs from broccoli, an avocado, a green salad, and some cooked spinach. The total comes to seventy grams of carbohydrates, but twenty-five grams of that is in the form of fiber. That means you've eaten forty-five grams of net carbs for that day, which is below the upper limit for a ketogenic diet.

Now, we don't want the nonfibrous carbs you eat to spike your blood sugar, so we're going to stick with vegetables that grow above ground. In the previous chapter, I mentioned the ones that are especially low on the glycemic index, and so have only a slight effect on your blood sugar. Here they are again: spinach, bok choy, broccoli, asparagus, lettuce and other leafy greens, kale, celery, Brussels sprouts, seaweed, leeks, peppers, onions, watercress, cauliflower, green beans, snow peas, artichokes, cucumbers, zucchini, tomatoes, avocados, and olives.

So, to be clear:

No grains.

No starchy plants such as potatoes or starchy beans.

No sweet fruit (for now).

No refined sugar. None.

No sugary drinks. Nada.

No sugary syrups. Nope.

If you're insulin resistant, you may need to take in even fewer carbs. But we'll consider that later.

Lots of Fat

As the foundation of your diet, eat natural fats such as extra virgin olive oil, butter, heavy cream, full-fat sour cream, lard, tallow, coconut oil, and ghee (clarified butter). This part of the diet may feel downright decadent. You can put dollops of heavy cream or coconut oil into your coffee and your tea. Whip the cream if you want. You can even try butter in there. Some people love it. Just don't add sugar.

If you can afford it, get animal fats from organic and pasture-raised animals raised on natural diets. (For cows, that would be grass.) If this is too costly for you, then do whatever you can. Not everyone can afford to pay four to five times the price for foods on the chance that they have a health benefit. And that's fine. With a bit of trial and error, you should be able to find a grocery-buying strategy that your body thrives on, without breaking the bank.

One thing that may save you some money: You can forget

about paying more for things like extra-lean hamburger meat. Eat fatty meats. If you eat chicken, include the skin and the dark meat. Fish? Cook it with oil. Bacon? Keep the fat. Hamburger meat? Skip the 93 percent lean. Go for the 80 percent lean, which is 20 percent fat. Or even 73 percent lean if you can find it. Fry it in a skillet so you don't lose the fat. Do the same with steaks and sausage.

Eat eggs cooked in natural oils. *No egg-white omelets*. Eat the whole egg plus the fat it's cooked in.

You can eat high-fat plants such as avocados and olives, as well as nuts and seeds such as pecans, macadamia nuts, walnuts, sunflower seeds, flax seeds, pistachios, almonds, and no-sugar-added almond butter. And high-fat cheese. But not too much of any of these, since they also contain protein and some carbs. Peanuts, which are legumes, might be okay in small amounts, but it's best to avoid them for now, since they have more carbs than nuts do.

If you're like me, you'll think, *If low-carb is good, low-carb and low-fat must be better*. You'll be tempted to pick the fat off the bacon, to keep your protein too high relative to fat, to pull the greasy skin off the chicken and eat a skinless grilled chicken breast and feel virtuous doing it. Don't do that.

Or, maybe you're not like me, in which case you can just enjoy yourself.

Fats and Greens

Cook spinach, bok choy, celery, broccoli, kale, and other leafy greens in your favorite natural fat. For cooking, pick fats that are solid at room temperature, such as coconut oil or butter. Other oils oxidize at high temperatures, and you don't want that to happen.

Eat green salads with lots of extra virgin olive oil.

Avoid the manufactured "vegetable" oils that dominate the cooking oil section of grocery stores—soy, corn, safflower, cotton seed, and canola. Despite their "heart healthy" branding, the more we learn, the less reason we have to consume them. Here's just one of many reasons: In the amounts we consume them, they probably foster inflammation in our bodies by throwing off the balance of omega-3 and omega-6 oils.[2] They won't kill you in the short run unless you have a severe allergy to them. And if you eat out, you can't purge every trace of them from your diet. But the only good argument in their favor is that they are cheap. The claim that they're healthier than natural fats is false.[3]

You don't need to make weird, low-carb substitutes for potatoes, pasta, and bread. Fats, meats, and vegetables are actual foods that people eat. Focus on those for now.

That said, there are thousands of great recipes online for those following a "ketogenic diet," which is what this is. You can make some of these recipes to add variety. See endnotes for some good websites.[4] If you want some pasta or rice, get konjac-root noodles and frozen, "riced" cauliflower.

There are also some menu items at popular chain restaurants that fit this diet. Yes, finding them and not being tempted by, say, the buttery biscuits at Chick-fil-A is like walking through a minefield in which the mines have powerful magnets and you're wearing a metal vest. But if you need to grab food on the go once in a while, you can. Cheeseburgers with lots of veggies will work, for instance, as long as you skip the bun. At some point, the need to grab food on the go will be a much less urgent problem because your body will have learned to burn fat and go much longer between meals. But when the need does arise, it's helpful to have a plan that gets you past the thick-crust pizza and the three-bun Big Mac.

And remember, whether eating out or at home, it's not enough just to avoid lots of carbs. You also want to avoid too much pure protein, as with grilled chicken breast and canned tuna. If you eat these, mix them with natural fat.

You may have that US government food pyramid still stuck in your mind, as I do. So here's a new food pyramid to help you remember. The details vary, but this is spot on in broad outline—a great visual tool for deprogramming yourself from the USDA food pyramid's grain-happy, carb-crazy recommendations. Copy this and put it someplace near the food in your house.

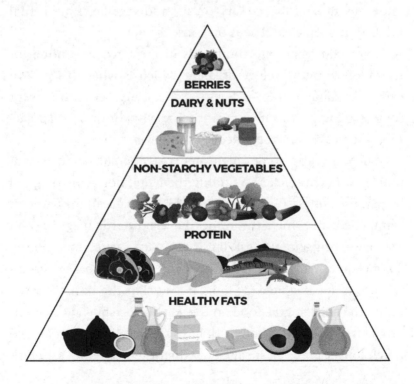

Artificial Sweeteners

What about artificial sweeteners, such as saccharin (Sweet'N Low), aspartame (NutraSweet), acesulfame potassium, and sucralose (Splenda)? Unfortunately, the controversy over these sweeteners makes it tough for nonspecialists to figure out what to do.

On the plus side, every official body that has studied their effects has concluded that they are safe. They are all GRAS according to the FDA—"generally regarded as safe." Also, they don't seem to do much directly to blood sugar, and most contain few, if any, calories. So, in that sense, they could be better than sugar for getting into ketosis. You might guess that using them as a substitute for sugar could help you lose body fat. But studies have had a hard time confirming this.

On the down side: They are all synthetic industrial products, and so none have been tested over the long haul of human history. They may be harmful, at least for some people, over decades of use. More relevant for our purposes: Some studies on humans, mice, and rats show that the sweeteners tested may raise insulin. One small study even linked sucralose (Splenda) to a higher blood sugar peak in obese patients than resulted from glucose.[5] Other studies have failed to show these effects.

Unfortunately, some studies suggest that sweeteners trigger an insulin response even if they don't affect blood sugar. Remember that insulin is the gatekeeper between our sugar-burning and fat-burning metabolisms. So the insulin response is a problem if your goal is to get into ketosis.

At the moment, two main theories suggest why it might be triggered. The first proposes that some or all these sweeteners change the balance in our gut bacteria (our "microbiome"), which play a major role in how we digest and respond to foods. This change might, in turn, make us more insulin resistant, which would lead to higher levels of blood sugar and insulin.

The other theory is that the sweet taste itself triggers an insulin response through taste receptors on our tongue.[6]

Both are plausible, and both may be true. I strongly advise being safe rather than sorry with artificial sweeteners. Avoid them as much as you can.

There's a third reason to avoid them, apart from how they may affect health and insulin: To become a lifestyle faster, you need to be metabolically flexible. And to do that, you need to cut way back on sweet foods. Not cut out entirely but cut way back. Not just for six weeks, but from now on.

It's much easier to do this if you reset your taste preferences. The more often intense, sweet flavors touch your tongue, the more you'll want them, and the less satisfied you'll be with less-sweet flavors. For instance, until I was in my thirties, I loved milk chocolate and couldn't stand the taste of dark chocolate. I still remember, as a kid, tossing out any dark chocolate candy that found its way into my Halloween stash.

As my palate matured, and I came to care about my health, I forced myself to eat dark chocolate—which has more of the healthy compounds called polyphenols than milk chocolate does. I now prefer it. Some time ago, I decided to go whole hog in working to reset my sweetness threshold. I cut out all drinks with artificial sweeteners, quit chewing sugar-free gum, and even bought the raw ingredients for a couple of pre-workout drinks I use, to avoid the sweet flavors. I now put these powders (all of which have a tart taste), in a big jug of water and drink it before I work out.

For a treat, I started eating squares of Trader Joe's 85 percent dark chocolate. Within a couple of weeks, my whole palate changed. Straight lime juice now tastes sweet to me, and grapefruit tastes as sweet as Dr. Pepper used to taste. I strongly recommend that you seize the chance, here at the beginning of your adaptation phase, to reset your taste preferences as well. There's really nothing to lose, and a lot to gain. My wife and I still eat 85 percent to 91 percent dark chocolate for a treat. If you eat just one or two squares of a bar, there's not much sugar in it, and you don't have to worry about artificial sweeteners.

That said, there are some sweeteners that we do use, especially in recipes. Stevia and sugar alcohols are processed, but both occur in nature and have been consumed by humans in some form for thousands of years. Truvía, which combines stevia and erythritol—the most benign of the sugar alcohols—is a good substitute for sugar in some recipes. But again, you should use these in moderation. For instance, you might save them for restrained use on feast days. The lower you can reset your preference for sweet flavors, the better.

Consume Lots of Water and Salt

Many people feel weird when they first shift into ketosis. As it happens, there's an easy way to avoid much or all of this: hydrate and keep your electrolytes up.

You should drink a lot of water. The "experts" often say eight eight-ounce glasses a day. I have been unable to find the scientific basis for this claim. Still, I'm a lean 170 pounds, highly active, and I drink more than twice that: about a gallon of water a day, not counting the water from foods, coffee, tea, and broth.

You should keep a water glass or water bottle full and near you at all times. If you want, add a slice of cucumber, lemon, or lime. At first, you might have to force yourself to drink when you're not really thirsty. But if you make it a habit, your body will start to remind you to drink more frequently.

Besides water, you need to bump up your intake of salt. Remember, your body is shedding water and sodium, so adding salt to your diet is not likely to spike your blood pressure. Add extra salt to your food. Put a pinch in your water. Drink chicken bouillon. You can even add salt to your coffee and tea. Don't knock it 'til you've tried it for a few weeks.

Getting enough salt is very important when switching into ketosis. When you're on a high-carb diet, such as the SAD, your body holds on to water—both your muscles and your kidneys play a role in this. When you ditch the carbs, though, out goes the water, and with it, electrolytes like sodium, potassium, and magnesium. Especially at first. Millions of people who have tried the low-carb Atkins diet over the last several decades felt flu-like symptoms. They thought dizziness, nausea, constipation, and headaches were just part of the process.

Sure, you should expect some trouble, such as carb craving, when switching your fuel source. Getting a hit of sugar provides a quick dopamine response: It feels like a little reward, but the feeling is fleeting and the craving returns quickly, since, as with any addictive thing you do over and over, it takes more and more of a sugar hit to enjoy the same pleasure. If you've spent many years feeding this response, you'll feel withdrawal symptoms when you stop.

There may also be moments during the shift when you feel weird. But there's no good reason for you to feel sick when switching into ketosis. In fact, you can avoid most if not all of the "keto flu"—dizziness, headaches, nausea—by drinking a lot of water and boosting your salt.[7] You might also take magnesium, potassium, and calcium supplements just to be on the safe side, at least for now.

Don't worry about the health risks of the extra salt, unless you have very high blood pressure. There's no evidence that dietary salt is bad for you otherwise.[8] Some of the healthiest and longest-lived populations on the planet, in places like Singapore and Japan, also eat the saltiest diets. For some groups, in fact, the more salt they eat, the lower their average blood pressure is. Whatever the details, there's no good reason to believe that salt is bad for us in general. If anything, a *low*-salt diet is a source of health problems.[9]

Hide the Scale

One final piece of advice for this first week: Hide the scale. You can weigh yourself before you start, but not at the end of the first week. Why? Because right now, the point isn't to lose weight. It's to teach your body to burn fat, on the way to being able to fast without it feeling like torture. If you need to lose body fat, that will happen over the next few weeks. You may lose weight this week, even as you increase your fat intake. But, as you might have guessed from the discussion of salt above, it will mostly be water weight. That's not trivial. If you lose seven pounds of water, your pants will fit more loosely around your waist. But if you have a weight problem and you weigh yourself, you might be tempted to extrapolate and assume the initial loss of weight will continue at the same pace from then on. In reality, the amount of water you retain will vary depending on whether you're in sugar-burning or fat-burning mode.

You will start losing body fat as a result of this process, but it's best not to confuse the big drop at the start of the transition with the normal loss of body fat that will follow for those with a lot of fat to lose. (The closer to an ideal weight you are, the more flexibility you'll have later to increase carbs.)

If You're Still Worried . . .

This plan, which involves eating a high-healthy-fat, low-carb, moderate-protein diet at the beginning, is based on solid science, years of clinical practice from informed physicians and nutritionists, and the testimony of thousands of self-experimenters, including me. For most people, it will work, and you'll be healthier for it. You'll also be one big step closer to a fasting lifestyle.

To embark on this journey, though, you'll have to ignore the busybodies who tell you you're clogging your arteries and killing yourself. Most people still believe that eating saturated fat causes coronary heart disease, cardiovascular disease, and strokes. (It doesn't.[10]) Reporters often tout studies that claim to show that low-carb or high-fat diets will kill you. There is now plenty of evidence that this just isn't true. But it's the rare person who can tackle the literature on the subject and explain it to know-it-alls while trying to learn how to fast.[11] If need be, just don't tell potential pests what you're doing.

But what if you still hear their voices inside your head? Are you still worried that eating all this fat will kill you? I get that. It took me years, plus self-experimenting and the reading of countless books and articles, to silence them in my own head. If it helps you rest more easily, you can get a complete blood panel beforehand, and then another a couple months after you've started the program.

You should make sure your doctor knows about fasting and ketogenic diets. And make sure the panel covers the following areas: First, test your hemoglobin (Hb) A1cs—this is a measure of your blood sugar level over a three-month period. It should be below 6 percent. Below 5 percent is better. (Note that in those already on a low-carb diet, A1c levels may be high because the red blood cells live longer. In those cases, the test renders a false positive. To find whether you have a problem or not, check fructosamine levels.)

Look especially at fasting blood glucose and hemoglobin A1cs. These should both go down between the first and second tests. Also look at blood triglycerides, which should go down as well.

Cholesterol is complicated. We were all taught to fear dietary cholesterol, even though most of the cholesterol in your system is produced by the liver itself. And in 2015, even the US government quit insisting that Americans needed to track total cholesterol in their diets.[12]

You've heard of HDL ("good") cholesterol and LDL ("bad") cholesterol. To simplify, an HDL is a little high-density lipoprotein submarine that transports waxy cholesterol from your blood to your liver, whereas an LDL is a low-density lipoprotein that ships cholesterol out of liver into the bloodstream. But even within LDL, there seem to be good and bad ones. The very small LDL particles are the ones that build up in artery walls that are inflamed or damaged. The larger, "fluffy" LDL particles don't tend to do that. So a newer test for LDL-p (*p* for "particle") now offers a more relevant measure. Get that if you can.

Total cholesterol is less important than the ratio of HDL to LDL. An HDL score of 50 is good. Above 70 is great. For triglycerides, under 100 (mg/dL) is good. Under 70 is great.

You can even do an NMR LipoProfile test, which gives more of the relevant data.*

Finally, you can have a CAC (coronary artery calcium) scan. This measures the actual calcium buildup in your coronary arteries, rather than trying to divine health from indirect and misleading numbers.[13] It's expensive, but it's a direct way to determine your cardiovascular health.

How to Prove You're Succeeding

If you're like me, you'll want to confirm that the strategy is working—that you really are switching your body into fat-burning mode. It would be nice to measure insulin directly, but that's difficult and expensive. Second best is to measure whether your blood sugar is staying on the low side of normal and your body is converting fat to ketones and burning them for fuel. The good news is that there are some inexpensive ways to do both, but that does not mean they are as simple as taking your temperature. You have to test either your urine or your blood. (See appendix 3 for details.)

---

* See more details on this webpage: https://www.ketogenic-diet -resource.com/blood-test-results.html.

WARNINGS AND DISCLAIMERS

1. Are you a child, severely underweight, pregnant, or nursing? Then you probably shouldn't fast. Do you have type 1 or 2 diabetes, take hormones, have metabolic problems or an eating disorder? If so, check with your doctor about fasting. You should find a doctor who knows about fasting and ketogenic diets, beyond what he or she picked up in the lounge in medical school. (You can find a list of such doctors at: www.ketogenicdocs.com.) Myths and prejudices are as common among physicians and nutritionists as they are in the general public.

2. If you have severely high blood pressure, talk to your doctor.

3. I'm not a physician, so you should not take what follows as medical advice.

4. I'm not saying that this is the only healthy way to fast or to eat.

5. I think this method is an excellent one for most people most of the time. Otherwise, I wouldn't recommend it. But humans are complicated, so your mileage may vary.

6. I don't propose a vegan or vegetarian diet, but I know there's more than one path to the fasting lifestyle (which is our goal). When I was thirty, I ate a very low-fat, high-protein, high-complex-carb diet. I was as fit as I've ever been. (I was also hungry all the time and found fasting very hard.) The Okinawans are famously healthy, even though for decades they've eaten a high-carb diet.

7. To keep this book from becoming inaccessible, I often provide technical references in the endnotes. If you want to do more research on a subject, check the notes.

9

Fasting for Discipline, Sacrifice, and Holiness

Our plan is designed to ease you into fasting. Still, I doubt you'll forget that it's a sacrifice. When you start to fast, you'll feel hunger. Let this serve to remind you that one reason you should fast is to discipline your natural appetites. To overcome temptations and addictions. To put your body's appetites under the control of your will, rather than leaving them to habit and autopilot. To become holy.

In his first letter to the church at Corinth, the apostle Paul wrote, "Athletes exercise self-control in all things; they do it to receive a perishable wreath, but we an imperishable one. So I do not run aimlessly, nor do I box as though beating the air; but I punish my body and enslave it, so that after proclaiming to others I myself should not be disqualified" (1 Cor. 9:25–27). He's not talking about being disqualified from a boxing contest. He's talking about the spiritual life. He's talking about his salvation.

Paul's point is not that our "animal nature" is the source of our sin. His point, rather, is that after the fall, our souls, our bodies, and our animal instincts are all fallen. They aren't separate compartments. You can't isolate your appetites to your biological self. If you don't get control of them, you might endanger your soul as well.

This idea of disciplining your natural appetites contradicts a secular myth: the Freudian theory of drives. We've all imbibed this idea whether we know it or not. Every urge, we imagine, becomes more and more intense—more *urgent*—until it's satisfied. Pop culture constantly claims that if teenagers don't have sex, for instance, they'll be repressed and have pent-up desires that will come out in destructive ways. Boys who don't have sex when they're sixteen will end up raping someone. Priests who don't get married will, just for that reason, molest prepubescent boys. A wife who doesn't blow up at her husband every time she gets irritated with him will have a nervous breakdown.

Of course, if you never deal with conflict in a healthy way and always avoid it, the fruits of that conflict may lead to worse problems later on. And we do have basic physical urges. You can't survive more than a few minutes without air or a few days without water. In such cases, our bodies are designed to want these ever more intensely the longer we go without them. Most of us can't hold our breath longer than ninety seconds.

But for many temptations, it's just not true that depriving yourself of them will make you want them all the more. Think of pornography for a porn addict, or alcohol for an alcoholic. Satisfying the urge to take one peek at a porn video, or one sip of vodka, doesn't satiate such people. It titillates the addicts and makes it even harder for them to stay on the wagon. Their pathway to success is to avoid even the hint of porn or alcohol.

Routine fasting is a great way to gain control over your

physical urges and impulses. Remember, fasting is not starvation. If you try to starve yourself when there's food around, at some point your willpower will give way to your body's need for food. (Unless you have severe anorexia, which is another matter.) Fasting, in contrast, is voluntary, controlled, and limited in time. If you practice it properly, it will become a habit. Keep at it, and it will become part of who you are. It will become a virtue. And the discipline you gain over food and eating can spill over into other areas of your life.

"Fasting," wrote St. Leo the Great, "gives strength against sin, represses evil desires, repels temptation, humbles pride, cools anger, and fosters all the inclinations of a good will even unto the practice of every virtue." Think about that for a minute. If Leo is right, then we can shape the state of our soul by what we do with our body. Somehow, our spirit is tied to our gastrointestinal system. That may seem weird. We're much more accustomed to thinking of physical disciplines, like working out, and spiritual disciplines, like prayer, as two separate things. But fasting reminds us that we aren't just bodies or souls. We are unities of body and soul. What affects the body affects the soul, and vice versa. This means that if we're properly disposed—unlike, say, the Pharisees whom Jesus criticized—then bodily sacrificing and suffering help make us more like Christ. This is one of the main purposes of fasting.

Suffering with Christ

Suffering is a part of the fallen human condition. And hunger is a form of suffering. The gospel tells us that God does not just observe suffering from a distance. He chose to save us, and redeem the creation, by entering fully into human suffering. In doing so, he also elevates our own suffering. "In bringing about the Redemption through suffering," St. Pope John Paul II wrote in his 1984 apostolic letter *Salvifici Doloris* explaining the power of "salvific suffering," "Christ has also raised human suffering to the level of the Redemption. Thus each man, in his suffering, can also become a sharer in the redemptive suffering of Christ."[1]

The terms "salvific" or "redemptive suffering" makes some folks uneasy. That's because it seems to suggest that we can save ourselves by our own good works. But the Church has denounced that idea ever since it was first suggested by Pelagius in the fifth century AD. We are saved by God's grace through the redemption Christ has made possible through his life, death, and resurrection. This is basic Christianity.

It doesn't follow, though, that we are excluded from this process. The New Testament clearly teaches just the opposite. Christ tells his disciples to take up their crosses daily. His yoke is easy and his burden is light, he tells us. But it is a yoke and a burden, and we are supposed to carry it.

According to St. Peter, you are supposed to "rejoice in so far as you share Christ's sufferings" (1 Pet. 4:13). Let that sink in. Peter is not just saying we should rejoice when we suffer for following Christ. Somehow, you and I are supposed to *share* Christ's sufferings.

What does that mean? Apologist Dave Armstrong puts it nicely:

> *I think it has to do with God involving us in His work all down the line. We know that He saves us by grace alone, yet we cooperate in that (also by His grace), to such an extent that*

St. Paul can say that "we are God's fellow workers" (1 Cor. 3:9)
and that we are "Working together with him" (2 Cor. 6:1);
indeed He tells us to "work out your own salvation . . . for God
is at work in you" (Phil. 2:12–13).[2]

We don't save ourselves. But our participation in Christ's sufferings is a key part of our salvation. God did not choose to save us with a distant, mere formal act. Though his own work would be enough to save us, he meant to take up our own suffering in his plan of salvation.

If you're still skeptical, look at a few more passages from Paul's letters, with emphasis added. Read them carefully, as if for the first time. And remember, Paul has been called the Apostle of Grace:

. . . fellow heirs with Christ, provided we suffer with him in
order that we may also be glorified with him (Rom. 8:17).

For as we share abundantly in Christ's sufferings, so
through Christ we share abundantly in comfort too. If we are
afflicted, it is for your comfort and salvation; and if we are
comforted, it is for your comfort, which you experience when
you patiently endure the same sufferings that we suffer. Our
hope for you is unshaken; for we know that as you share in our
sufferings, you will also share in our comfort (2 Cor. 1:5–7).

We are . . . always carrying in the body the death of Jesus,
so that the life of Jesus may also be manifested in our bodies.
For while we live, we are always being given up to death for

Jesus's sake, so that the life of Jesus may be made visible in our mortal flesh" (2 Cor. 4:8–11).

I have been crucified with Christ; it is no longer I who live, but Christ who lives in me . . . (Gal. 2:20).

Henceforth let no one trouble me; for I bear on my body the marks of Jesus (Gal. 6:17).

. . . that I may know him and the power of his resurrection, and may share his sufferings, becoming like him in his death . . . (Phil. 3:10).

And finally, perhaps to confound all our expectations, Paul wrote to the church at Colossi,

Now I rejoice in my sufferings for your sake, and in my flesh I complete what is lacking in Christ's afflictions for the sake of his body, that is, the church (Col. 1:24).

So close is Paul's suffering with Christ's that the apostle can speak of himself suffering for the Church, even completing "what is lacking in Christ's afflictions." How does that work?

Well, first, remember that Paul knew that whatever good works were happening in him with his cooperation were in fact works of Christ. They have merits because they are Christ's works. And logically, though Christ could work in and through Paul, he could not at the same time be Paul. So that part—Paul freely suffering as well—would be lacking in Christ's afflictions while on the earth. It's lacking not because Christ could not have done it all on his own, but because, from the beginning, he chose to include not just his own sufferings, but ours as well. Who are we to argue with him? He is God, and we are not.

This is why Christians have every reason, when we suffer, to "offer up our suffering" for others. Our suffering is taken up into the redemptive suffering of the Lord. That includes our fasts.

Penance

Just as we can offer our suffering through Christ as a sacrifice for others, we can also offer our suffering for repentance. Personal and communal penance has long been one of the uses of fasting—and one of the many that has fallen into disuse. But that may be changing. In September 2018, four Augustinian priests in Long Island, New York, announced a twenty-five-day "communal penance":

> *As a response to the horrific revelations not only of the abuse of children, but also of seminarians and priests by priests, bishops and cardinals which have surfaced, we . . . have decided to undertake a communal penance of fasting and abstinence in reparation for these sins of others. From 4 September until the Anticipatory Mass of 29 September (the Feast of the Holy Archangels), we will take only water and a modest vegetarian diet.*[3]

Let's pray that these tiny embers of fasting, provoked by scandal among Catholic bishops, will become a wildfire consuming sin and corruption among Christians and ushering in a new spirit of repentance that fills our whole lives. As St. Pope Paul VI explains in his apostolic letter on fasting and penance, "Thus the task of bearing in his body and soul the death of the Lord affects the whole life of the baptized person at every instant and in every aspect."[4]

Holiness

After baptism, the Christian life is meant to be one of progress. You should be in a state of being constantly transformed into the likeness of Christ. This is not a matter of trying to save yourself, but of surrendering to Christ, who wants to work inside you through the Holy Spirit. He won't force this on you. You have to cooperate. In his Sermon on the Mount, Jesus says, "Blessed are those who hunger and thirst for righteousness, for they will be filled" (Matt. 5:6). We don't want just to be declared righteous. We should want to be *made* righteous.

Peter reminds us that we are to be holy as God is holy (1 Pet. 1:16). That's not easy. Paul goes so far as to describe this process, starting at baptism, as one of dying with Christ, and then rising with him. "I have been crucified with Christ," he writes to the church in Rome, "and I no longer live, but Christ lives in me. The life I now live in the flesh I live by faith in the Son of God, who loved me and gave himself for me" (Gal. 2:20). This is such a common passage that many of us can recite it by memory. That makes it easy to miss how radical it is. Paul doesn't say that Christ is his co-pilot, or that Christ now lives with him and helps him get things done or carries him on the beach. He says, "I no longer live." Yes, this is hyperbole. Paul doesn't cease to exist, but still. He's clearly referring to his old self apart from Christ, trapped in sin and compounded by self-righteousness because he observed the Jewish laws so well.

Christ died to save Paul, you, and me from our sins—and also to transform our very being—if we will let him. This is the pursuit of holiness. To be holy is not just to be sanctified, but to be "set apart" from the baser things of the world. And since eating is a biological imperative, fasting is a simple way to set yourself apart. It allows you to detach yourself temporarily from one of your most basic biological needs—for both spiritual and physical benefit. It also allows you to take a break from our pervasive consumer culture, which has a bottomless appetite. This is one path both to greater holiness but also to greater freedom. As St. Pope John Paul II put it during a Lenten message in 1979, "Going without things is to free oneself from the slaveries of a civilization that is always urging people on to greater comfort and consumption."[5] That's true whether we're talking about the newest smartphone, a larger flat-screen TV, or a scrumptious meal that we want but can do without.

WEEK TWO

10

16/8 Time-Restricted Eating

In week one of our plan, you cut way back on carbs, moderated proteins, and boosted fats in your diet to switch your body from the crests-and-falls pace of sugar burning to slow and steady fat burning. In week two, you'll break the habit of eating throughout your waking hours. Instead, you'll start to restrict the window of time in which you eat. This will make your daily fast longer than it has been.

You Already Fast

Huh? Why did I write "longer than it has been"? Because, as we've already noted, you've fasted every day of your life. To fast is simply to abstain from food. When you're sleeping, you're not eating. So, if you finish your last meal at 7:00 p.m., and don't eat again until 7:00 a.m. the next morning, you've survived a twelve-hour fast. Good job!

We don't think much about this because we're sleeping most of the time. Also, we don't really enter a fasting state until several hours after our last meal, since our body spends several hours processing the food. We should thank God that we need to sleep eight hours or so. Otherwise, few of us would ever really enter a fasting state. And our bodies would be the worse for it.

As long as you're running on sugar, though, you need to eat early and often. The ups and downs of blood sugar and insulin will see to that. And this pattern keeps your blood sugar and insulin levels above the range that allows your body to really use its fat stores. That, in turn, makes true fasting hard to do.

Once you're running mainly on ketones rather than glucose, though, there's no good reason to eat every few hours. You can lengthen your usual nightly fast without your brain and body going into panic mode.

Delay Breakfast

You may be thinking, *Oh no. He's going to say I should skip breakfast, isn't he?* Well, yes, sort of. I understand the fear. I preached the gospel of oatmeal and egg-white omelets for years. Skipping breakfast, I thought, would slow down my metabolism and cost me lean muscle. But as we noted earlier, that idea is a myth. When your body first moves into a fasted state, it kicks up its metabolism and boosts growth hormone. That gives you energy, and helps your body save muscle and burn fat.

There's no biological need to eat right after you get up in the morning. In fact, just before you wake up, your cortisol goes up and your liver releases sugar into your bloodstream. Your body has already supplied your short-term energy needs without you needing to throw down a smoothie at 7:15 a.m. Try a couple of glasses of water instead, and calorie-free coffee or tea if you drink them. Another benefit. Some research suggests that if you can avoid eating for an hour or two after waking, you'll sleep better. The theory is that when we eat right after we wake up, we set ourselves up for what is known as anticipatory waking: You wake up because your body associates waking with eating yummy food, usually sugar-rich carbs. Break that link and you may find yourself sleeping better.

In fact, you don't *need* to eat in the morning at all. This is a custom, not a necessity. That doesn't mean you have to skip breakfast. After all, your first meal of the day will be breakfast—it will *break your fast*—no matter when you eat it. If you like "breakfast food," there's nothing to stop you from eating bacon and eggs in the afternoon.

So, think of this part of our plan as *delaying* breakfast. It's called time-restricted eating or intermittent fasting. You will just limit the range of time during the day when you eat all of your meals. If you've spent decades eating six or more little meals a day and eating from the moment your head leaves the pillow until just before it returns to your pillow, it might be hard at first. But remember that as recently as the 1970s, most folks ate just three meals a day. I'm old enough to remember that routine as a small child. If you ate breakfast at 8:00 a.m. and finished dinner at 6:00 p.m., and didn't have a bedtime snack, you would go thirteen or fourteen hours without food every day.

Eating exactly three meals was also just a custom—though for people of European ancestry, it may go back in some form to the Middle Ages.[1] But the big breakfast and dinner custom is a recent American thing. Cereal as a breakfast staple owes its origins to Will Keith Kellogg and John Harvey Kellogg, who introduced cornflakes in 1897 as a "healthy alternative," based on the vegetarianism they practiced as Seventh Day Adventists.[2] Did you know you owe your breakfast-eating habits to Seventh Day Adventist beliefs?

Normally, we don't need to eat three meals. But if you're wedded to that, fine. Just squeeze them into an eight-hour window for this stage of our forty-six-day plan. The key here is the sixteen-hour daily fast, which will start to teach your body to burn fat. Plus, this daily balance between fasting and feeding states has health benefits. It helps keep our bodies insulin sensitive—that's good—by allowing our insulin levels to drop for a good chunk of time every day. If you're also in ketosis, the benefit will be even greater. So this week you'll start to combine the power of ketosis with time-restricted eating.

The Sixteen-Hour Fast

I presume you already fast for about eight hours at night and eat over a sixteen-hour period during the day. If so, then for the next week, just flip that. Pick an eight-hour window in which you eat as much as you did last week with the same mix of low carbs, some protein, and a lot of fat. For the other sixteen hours, fast from all food—that is, from calories. Drink lots of water (and coffee or tea if you like) throughout the day. You can also sip warm bouillon. (Just make sure it has very few calories, and check for weird additives.)

This daily rhythm is the so-called 16/8 method popularized several years ago by Martin Berkhan at Lean Gains (www.lean gains.com). It's also the method I follow on most days.

Of course, your body will *expect* food at fixed times. Your stomach will growl around lunch- and dinnertime just as surely as Pavlov's dog salivated when he heard the bell ring. You'll have to resist these little body signals, such as a gurgling stomach. But if you've followed the rules from week one, you won't feel desperate for food. And at some point, even these tempting signals will diminish.

For me, the easiest way to do a sixteen-hour fast is to delay my first meal of the day. For instance, I may eat breakfast at 1:00 p.m. and then stop eating at 9:00 p.m. There's nothing magical about that though. You may prefer to start at noon and end at 8:00 p.m. Or, depending on your schedule, you may pick different time windows on different days. That's fine too. Do whatever works best for you. The main thing is to eat all of your food for the day within an eight-hour period. Many people, this author included, find it easier to sleep if they eat most of their carbs later in the day. I often eat green vegetables, as well as a big salad with lots of olive oil, at my last meal.

On Sunday, you have a mini-feast. Expand your feeding-time window if you want. Perhaps eat a handful of blueberries, strawberries, or blackberries, or a couple of squares of 85 percent dark chocolate in place of some vegetables. Don't go crazy. You're still in the transition phase. Your body will be only too happy to drop out of its fat-burning mode at this point. Still, you can do something to mark the weekly mini-feast day and remind your body that all is not lost.

Sixteen hours may sound like a long time to go, but it's really not. Before my wife, Ginny, started fasting, she was sure that if she went sixteen hours without any food, she'd feel miserable. That's because, well, if she went more than a few hours without eating, she felt miserable. But after she learned about the effects of sugars and carbs, she started to adjust her diet keto-ward. Then, when she started to fast, it was no big deal. She now follows the 16/8 fast on most days. She reports far more "clarity and energy" when she does so.

Does she ever want to eat during the fast? Yes, but she no longer gets panicky and light-headed—symptoms she had long thought were signs of hypoglycemia. She's just hungry. Besides, she tells me, "the occasional pangs of hunger are a reminder for me to pray and to offer up to God my small suffering for others." That's good, because fasting and prayer go together.

11

Fasting for Better Prayer

Prayer and fasting have always been paired in Christian spirituality. Together they command the focus of your whole person—body, mind, and soul. The fasting lifestyle is about your physical and spiritual life. It reminds us that these two aspects of our being are not separate compartments.

If you're following the plan, you'll now be doing a real daily fast, even if you're netting the same amount of food per day. That means you'll have to resist low-level hunger pangs. You'll also have extra time in your day, because you'll spend less time preparing food and eating. What should you do? Pray. That includes mental prayer, spoken prayer, memorized prayers, and written prayers; prayers alone and prayers with your family or prayer group; spiritual reading; reading and studying Scripture. Are you not all that good at prayer? I would recommend a terrific book by the late Thomas Dubay, *Deep Conversion, Deep Prayer*.[1] Just read it and follow his advice. Other good books include *Beginning to Pray* by Anthony Bloom, and *Praying God's Word* by Beth Moore.

The Liturgy of the Hours

The fasting lifestyle should help you get in sync with the ups and downs of the Christian year. As God created the universe in six mysterious days, so our hours, and days, and weeks, recapitulate salvation history. There is one prayer discipline especially built for this tempo: The Divine Office or Liturgy of the Hours, also called the Breviary. If you need to amp up your prayer life and define your days with prayer, but aren't sure where to start, this is it.

The Divine Office ("office" is from the Latin word *opus*, meaning "work") has been part of Christian life in some form since the first century.

Its origin story is complex and would take us too far afield to trace here. But it helps to have a little history. The Divine Office takes up the ancient Jewish tradition of a daily sacrifice, plus morning and evening prayers. As the psalmist says: "Evening and morning and at noon/I utter my complaint and moan/and he will hear my voice" (Ps. 55:17). Indeed, until the temple of Jerusalem was destroyed in AD 70, prayers were offered in the morning, evening, and nighttime.

And it wasn't just non-Christian Jews. Acts records in passing Peter and John going to the temple in Jerusalem "at the hour of prayer" (Acts 3:1).

The *Didache*, written around the first century AD, advised the faithful to pray the Lord's Prayer (Our Father) three times a day, and this became part of the pattern.

Early Christianity spread throughout the cities of the Roman Empire. And it wasn't long before bells rang during fixed hours of the day in these cities. This helped citizens coordinate their work and organize their daily communal, prayers.

Christians knew that Paul had written to the church at Thessalonica to "pray without ceasing" (1 Thess. 5:17). Early monks did their best to apply this literally. They soon figured out that it took a group effort.[2]

These prayers—fixed to the hours of the day—became the structure for monastic life that continues to this day (along with daily Mass and Scripture readings). Early monastics saw the psalms as perfect prayers and so resolved to pray them verbatim. That's why the Divine Office is built around the psalms. It also includes other short readings from Scripture, short prayers, and the hymns spoken by Zechariah, Mary, and Simeon in the gospels. The morning and evening hours include the Lord's Prayer.[3]

The Divine Office, or Liturgy of the Hours, isn't just for priests and monks.[4] As with fasting, millions of laypeople pray the Office as well. Indeed, it is often called the "prayer of the whole people of God." So why do so few laypeople participate? Probably because the whole thing looks imposing and complex. Yes, it does include prayers, which you memorize if you stick with the routine for a couple of months. But there's also a complicated cycle of psalms, hymns, antiphons, short prayers, and scripture readings. Overlaid on top of that are various and sundry saint days and feast days, which can land on different days of the week. And overlaid on top of that is the annual liturgical calendar, with its three separate year cycles.

Early on, monks would need several different volumes to keep up. It was such a problem that around the eleventh century a master list of the Divine Office was developed, called the *breviarium*. This is why the books containing the Divine Office are called breviaries. So, if you were wondering, Liturgy of the Hours, the Divine Office, and the Breviary refer to the same thing. Still more complexity!

Before Gutenberg introduced the printing press in Europe, ordinary folks could not afford to own the texts needed to pray the Breviary. These days, we don't have that excuse. Still, even if it doesn't cost much in terms of dollars, most laypeople find the Liturgy of the Hours intimidating. I started praying it by good luck. Years ago, before I became Catholic, I took a week-long retreat at a monastery in Illinois. For a full week, I experienced the prayers chanted by the monks. I just followed what they were doing. The monks weren't too chatty, but they were kind enough to write instructions on a chalkboard for the uninitiated men sitting in the back of the chapel.

What do you do if you can't make it to the local monastery every morning and evening? For a long time, the easiest way to pray the Breviary on your own was to buy the four-volume set. Unfortunately, it's bulky and expensive (around $150). There's a less expensive single-volume version that has the complete morning and evening prayers but alas, it requires a separate annual guide, since some of the details change from year to year. And it comes with a rainbow of separate colored ribbons, since you have to flip to different sections throughout a single hour. (It doesn't really take an hour. More like fifteen minutes.) I wanted to pray the morning, evening, and night prayers, though, so I got a single-volume version in 2008 and read several articles to figure out how to do it. The process became second nature after a few months. Still, it's hardly surprising that most people don't have the patience for this.

Fortunately, there are now shortcuts. One is the terrific publication called *Magnificat*, which comes as both a monthly print magazine and an app. It combines shortened morning, evening, and nighttime prayers, with the daily Mass readings and first-rate classical and contemporary spiritual writings. These are arranged intuitively and don't require guidebooks and color-coded ribbons. My wife has subscribed for years.

Another, even more affordable shortcut: Just download the free (!) smartphone app called iBreviary. It provides all the right prayers at the right time in a simple order. All you have to do is tap, scroll, and pray.

If you want something on the Protestant side of the aisle, visit www.anglicanbreviary.net and explore the Resources tab.[5] If you compare the Anglican and Catholic versions, you will notice that they look a lot alike. That is because both are drawing upon practices common since early Christianity.

So now you have resources to simplify matters. You also have more time on your hands because you don't spend all day eating. After all, we can really only focus on one thing at a time. As Peter Kreeft observes, "In order to create time to pray, we must destroy time to do something else. We must kill something, refuse something, say no to something."[6] When you say no to food, you should say yes to prayer. If you fast regularly, you really don't have a good excuse not to pray at least the morning and evening prayers. Make it a fixed part of your fasting routine. At least try it for a few weeks. If you stick with it, it will change your prayer life, your relationship to time, and your relationship with God.

WEEK THREE

Three Days with the 20/4 Routine

After a few days of eating in an eight-hour window, you may find that it's not as hard as you thought it would be, since your body has started to use fat from your diet and even from your body for energy. The longer you do this, the easier it will be for you. Trust me.

Now, in the third week, you will limit your feeding window even more—to four hours. That is, eat all your meals during a four-hour period. I do this regularly two to three times a week, usually on Monday, Wednesday, and Friday. You can try different times or pick a slot that works best for you—5:00 p.m. to 9:00 p.m. works best for me. But some people like to start earlier in the day. Whichever one you do, you will now have a daily fasting window of twenty consecutive hours. Do this for as many days as you can, but for at least three of the seven days.

You don't need to try to restrict calories. In theory, you can eat as much as you were eating before. But you may eat less. It's hard to pack three full meals into four hours when you're eating lots of fat and very few carbs except for green veggies. Don't force yourself to eat more once you start to feel full.

Force-feeding is rarely a good idea. If anything, slow down as soon as you feel your stomach swelling.

You'll feel full when you reach the volume of a regular meal. If you stop, you may feel hungry an hour or so later. And if you still haven't eaten a full day's calories after your second meal, the same thing may happen an hour or so after that. This is what happens when I eat in a four-hour window. I'm not sure why. My best guess is that our bodies have a natural set point, which calls for an average number of calories. When you restrict the time during the day when you eat, the signals of hunger and satiety adjust to try to get your body back on track.

Again, don't forget to drink lots of water and perhaps salty bouillon. If you like coffee or tea, that's fine too. Just don't add calories to them during the fasting window.

On Sunday, ease up on the fasting since it's a feast day. Expand your feeding-time window to twelve hours. In place of some veggies perhaps eat a handful of blueberries, strawberries, or blackberries, half of a medium-size pink grapefruit, or a couple of squares of 85 percent dark chocolate. Don't worry that this modest feast is all you'll ever get. Later, your body will have a firmer grip on its fat-burning powers. But at this stage you're still in transition. Your body will be only too happy to drop out of its fat-burning mode and take on several pounds of water. Still, do something to mark the weekly mini-feast day. You have something to celebrate.

Why Fasting Isn't an Attack on Your Body

You've already seen some of the scientific evidence that fasting is not bad for your health. Still, if you've heard stories about the ascetic extremes of early Christians, you may find it hard to shake the impression that fasting is still, in some sense, an attack on the body. If so, then fasting, or some kinds of fasting, would contradict Christian belief itself.

A Starving Monk, Whipping Himself

We all have a mental picture—fed by Hollywood—of a medieval monk, lashing himself to bits. We can see in our minds his hollow and ashen face, his ribs protruding from his side, his malnourishment, all to "mortify" and subdue his sinful flesh. If he succeeds, he will die of hunger or disease, and will finally be free from the prison of his body.

My own mental image is slightly different, but so specific that I was sure it must have been formed by a movie. Sure enough, I recently stumbled upon the source. In the classic comedy film

Monty Python and the Holy Grail—which I saw several times in junior high and high school—there's a scene of a group of seven monks wearing dark brown habits with hoods pulled forward to cover their eyes. They are marching slowly through a stereotypical medieval village, with smoke in the air, hay at their feet, and the lowing of cattle in the background. They are singing a Gregorian chant, over and over: *"Pies Iesu Domine / Dona eis requiem."* "Blessed Lord Jesus, grant them rest." And on the last beat of the second line, in unison, they bang themselves on the head with a board!

Sure, it's funny, and it captures the stereotype. But like every stereotype, it distorts as much as it clarifies. I'm not saying that no such monk ever lived, and died an early death from overly zealous fasting and mortification of the flesh. The truth is, the self-tormented monk isn't entirely a Hollywood fiction. Some fasting among some Christians inclined in that direction. In such cases, they were veering dangerously close to the earliest heresy of Gnosticism.

What I am saying is that such extreme practices contradict the balanced *Christian* view of the spiritual life. They contradict the Christian picture of what it means to be human.

A Unity of Body and Soul

We are, each of us, unities of matter and spirit, body and soul. We are made from the dust of the earth and the breath of God. We're neither mere matter nor ghosts trapped in bodies. We're bodily persons. We are created good, but we are now fallen—body and soul. This idea is part of the basic deposit of Christian theology. Everything else we say about men and women must fit with it.

The fact that we are bodily persons bears directly on how God has acted in history. If you don't know what man is, you won't understand what it meant for God to *become* man. God came to earth, not as an angel or a ghost, but as a man. Yes, a man who represented every man and woman who will ever live. But he was—is—also a unique man who lived at a specific time and place. To make the point crystal clear, Christians from very early on have said that God became incarnate. That is, *he became flesh.* In his body, he died for our sins. He rose—bodily—from the dead. He ate breakfast with his disciples after the resurrection. Forty days later, he ascended, body and all, into heaven. His tomb was empty.

As St. Paul tells us in his first letter to the Corinthians, this is why we have hope in the life to come. We look forward not just to a vaporous existence as souls in heaven, but as people with new bodies (1 Cor. 15:35–55). In a new heaven and new earth. Yes, as Paul explains, these bodies will be far more glorious than our present bodies. He compares our present and resurrected bodies to a kernel of grain and the subsequent plant grown from it. But the new body is a real body. If you're picturing it as a shimmery patch of thin fog, ask yourself, is that really what Paul's image of a seed and the plant it becomes would lead one to expect of our glorified bodies? Of course it isn't.

Thus, we believe, as the ancient creed puts it, both in the life everlasting *and* the resurrection of the body.

Does it seem like I'm saying the same thing over and over with slightly different words? That's because I am. This truth—that we are a unity of matter and spirit, material and immaterial, body and soul—bears endless repeating, because it is so easy to get wrong. It's so easy to fixate on either the physical or spiritual side, when the path of truth requires us to hold both together.

Gnosticism? None for Me, Thanks

In practice, what this means is that spiritual disciplines that harm or revile the body are not fully Christian, because they deny the goodness of the body and, by extension, the goodness of God's physical creation. No Christian fast should ever be like this.

The first heresy of the Christian era made just this mistake. Gnosticism, a form of which the Apostle John may already have been fighting when he wrote his gospel, cut an unbridgeable chasm between body and soul, between spirit and matter. Gnostics taught an extreme dualism between matter and spirit. Matter, they thought, was evil, and spirit was good.

Marcion (c. AD 85 – c. AD 160) is a classic if eccentric champion of this view. He drank deeply from the well of pagan Greek philosophy, which lacked the balanced biblical view of the human person. Greek philosophy was not the handmaid of theology for Marcion but rather its master. After reading the Old Testament, he concluded that the God Jesus spoke of could not be the same God. There must, he posited, be two "Gods." One was the vengeful, jealous tribal deity of the Hebrews who fashioned the material world. The other was a spiritual, all-loving and forgiving God who utterly transcended the material world and who alone was worthy of worship.

It should be no surprise that Marcion and other Gnostics had to redefine—that is, deny—the incarnation and resurrection of Jesus. After all, why would God, a great spirit, assume evil matter? Marcion had his own preferred canon, which excluded the Old Testament, but included ten of Paul's letters and some selected passages from Luke's gospel that didn't contradict his views.

Every major heretic motivated the early Church toward greater doctrinal clarity, and Marcion was no exception. He was a major catalyst for the Church to define the true canon, which excluded texts tainted by the Gnostic heresy.

Some Gnostics reasoned that they should treat the body as the enemy and do whatever they could to degrade it. Other Gnostics went to an opposite extreme. They held that what you do with your body doesn't really matter because the material realm doesn't really matter. These Gnostics might engage in gluttony and all manner of sexual perversion, because such acts touched only the body, not the soul.

Thus the heretic's hatred for the body, Anthony Esolen writes, "bears twins in evil. We have either a Manichean loathing of the body as source and sink of wickedness, made by an evil sub-deity; or a gnostic antinomianism, lending us free rein to pant after bodily pleasures of all kinds."[1]

Even Christians who rejected full-blown Gnosticism still might not get the balance right. The Church Father Origen (c. AD 184–254) stands as a warning to all of us. As a teenager, he was not just willing to die for his faith (as his father did) but sought it out—only to be persuaded by his mother not to do so. Throughout his career, he was given to extreme bouts of asceticism. He did not just abstain from all alcohol. He was a strict vegetarian who often fasted for dangerously long periods of time. He wore no shoes and slept on the floor. Eusebius, the first Church historian, reports that Origen even castrated himself. Some scholars dispute that,[2] but his general behavior was extreme enough to give the claim legs. He took a dim view of the body and the material creation. A fasting lifestyle that is robustly Christian must rest on firmer foundations. And, I'm happy to say, it can and should rest on less troubling foundations. Indeed, it should rest on encouraging ones.

Yes, God expects us to sacrifice. Indeed, he sometimes calls us to suffer severe pain, even to sacrifice our lives for a greater good. History tells us that every apostle suffered physical persecution for his faith, with all but one of them dying for the faith. As Jesus tells his disciples in the Gospel of John, "Greater love has no man than this, that a man lay down his life for his friends" (John 15:13). Now, most of us won't face this level of persecution even if we live very bold lives for Christ. The normal Christian life isn't about holding steady in front of a literal firing squad. It's about the daily walk, about subduing our sinful desires, and training our bodies, minds, and souls to know God, to glorify him, and to enjoy him forever. Fasting is one means to that end. It's not about degrading our bodies or treating them as the taproot of evil.

The Church councils, and the creeds that emerged from them in the fourth and fifth centuries, defended and defined Christ's full divinity and humanity.[3] These provided guardrails to prevent Christian spirituality from descending into the rejection of the body so common in Eastern religion.

Still, by our lax modern standards, almost any robust practice from the Middle Ages is bound to look extreme. And some really were extreme. A few of these may have been miraculously assisted and deeply ordered in the divine will, as was Moses's forty-day fast from both food and water (physically impossible without a miracle). Others were simply disordered and misguided.

But there are also outliers. Take the phenomenon exhibited by some women in the Middle Ages, called "miraculous lack of appetite" (anorexia mirabilis). Some of these women became saints, and one, St. Catherine of Siena (1347–1380), has even been declared a Doctor of the Church. She entered religious life as a young teenager and went so far as to renounce all food for years except for the Eucharist. And she didn't even have access to daily Mass.

Some modern scholars have tried to tie this to the modern condition of anorexia nervosa. Did St. Catherine and others like her suffer from a psychological disorder, and just dress it in Christian terms? I used to think that, but the longer I've studied this, the more convinced I've become that this charge is not just anachronistic. It's also patronizing, since it fails to consider what St. Catherine in particular said she was doing. She didn't write anguished letters about her thick ankles and the cellulite on her thighs before entering into this discipline. She didn't imagine that she was overweight when in fact she was gaunt. She was a spiritual force of nature, and a profound thinker to boot.

In her definitive study of food and women in the Middle Ages, Caroline Walker Bynum points out the obvious difference between anorexia mirabilis and anorexia nervosa. "The twentieth-century girl refused food in order to assert control over her body," she writes; "the fourteenth-century saint refused food in order to eat God and feed her fellow sinner."[4]

If we knew nothing else about St. Catherine but her miraculous lack of appetite, we might deem her disordered. But we know more than this. We know that St. Catherine, like

St. Francis, was given the great, terrible, supernatural gift of the stigmata—wounds on the body akin to the wounds from Christ's crucifixion. We can surmise that her "miraculous lack of appetite," like the stigmata, was also a rare and supernatural gift. It went far beyond merely lacking an appetite for food. Why? Because, even if she had received the Eucharist every day, that would not be enough to naturally sustain a person. In the natural order of things, most people would starve to death within a couple of months. If she survived on, say, fifty calories a day for years on end, we must conclude that God sustained her directly.

Because it was a very rare miracle, however, hers is not a method Christians as a whole can emulate. We should no more take it as the norm for fasting than a Christian baker should take Jesus's feeding of the five thousand as the normal way Christians get bread.

We should judge the deeds of saints by the fruits they bear. Here is one fruit of St. Catherine's life: She helped the Church recover from one of the Church's darkest moments. During St. Catherine's time, the pope—you know, the *bishop of Rome*—was actually exiled in Avignon, France. No doubt many faithful Christians at the time thought the Church was on its last legs. But they were wrong. The Holy Spirit, working through a fully yielded vessel, renewed the Body of Christ on earth. And this despite the fact that St. Catherine lived a mere thirty-three years on this earth—just as Christ did.

Perhaps, to vanquish some great evils, only spiritual superpowers will suffice—stigmata, sleeping on the hard floor, consecrated virginity, and surviving supernaturally on nothing but the Eucharist. In such extreme cases, we should resolve to let

God do what he wants to do. Sometimes it involves spiritual superheroes.

Of course, some took the "mortification of the flesh" to dangerous lengths—with no hint of a miraculous mandate. In the eleventh century, Benedictine monk St. Peter Damien, a great soldier against Church corruption, practiced flagellation as a form of penance. The practice, a small imitation of the scourging Christ suffered before his crucifixion, soon spread to other monasteries around Europe. Later, when plagues and famines were sweeping the continent, so-called flagellants brought the practice into cities.

What started as a private act of monastic penance soon became a spectacle. Whole processions of the flagellants became common in cities, and over time went off the rails. Some flagellants began to preach that one could wipe away one's sins through these public whipping sessions, at which point the pope condemned them (1261). When other extreme forms of self-flagellation emerged in the Middle Ages, the Church condemned that as well.

Still, the private practice of self-flagellation continued for centuries for penance and discipline. For instance, Augustinian monk Martin Luther (yes, that Martin Luther) still used the practice long after 1517. And it continues as a private practice to the present day.

Body and Soul United Together

Too much Christian thinking on fasting, even now, is limited to asceticism, self-denial, and "mortification of the flesh." Some authors imply that a fast that makes you feel better and more energetic wouldn't be a sacrifice, and so wouldn't be a real fast! When I wrote a series touting all the benefits of fasting during Lent 2017, one reader accused me of *sacrilege* in the comments box. This is how a dilute Gnosticism manifests itself among pious Christians.

True Christian fasting, as Susan Mathews explains, "is not a pitting of the spirit against the flesh, but rather body and soul united together against sin, body and soul converted together to the Lord. The whole man must cooperate with God's grace. The whole man must love the Lord."[5]

In the same spirit, the great Orthodox theologian Alexander Schmemann wrote that true "Christian asceticism is a fight, not *against* but *for* the body."[6] A properly Christian fast should be for the whole person—body, mind, and soul.

14

Exercise for the Fasting Lifestyle

Most of this book is about eating and spiritual practices. But there are other important elements to a healthy lifestyle, including meaningful work, community, sleep, and exercise. We know that people who have a sense of purpose, have rich relationships, and get enough sleep and regular exercise have, on average, much healthier lives than those who don't.

I can't discuss all these matters without doubling the length of this book. But the benefits of exercise are so great, and complement the fasting lifestyle so well, that I would be remiss if I didn't include at least a primer. I can't customize a workout routine for you. But I can boil down the key principles and tips to keep in mind when you devise one.

First, let's debunk a myth. Far too many of us believe that working out by itself will cause us to lose weight—that is, to lose body fat. But this idea commits the same mistake we've seen over and over: It imagines that we can change one variable of our activity or metabolism without affecting the other. In fact, if you exercise, you'll probably be hungrier and need to eat more.

This is just good design. If you're regularly tearing muscle fibers by lifting weights, for instance, your body will need nutrients to repair and rebuild. If everything is working right, you'll get signals from your body to eat more. Every mom used to know that kids could "work up an appetite," but we forget this fact when we start thinking about diet and exercise.

Exercise does many important things, including changing our body composition, improving our health, and increasing both our insulin sensitivity and our mental acuity. That's why we should all exercise if we can. But remember: If you exercise, you'll want and need more food than you did before. Don't expect to offset a bad diet by working out.

Why You Should Exercise

You should exercise—that is, use your body to do work—because that's how God designed us. We're not supposed to sit around all day. To be more specific, we should exercise to maintain lean muscle mass and bone density and to keep our cardiovascular system in good working order. Resistance training is really crucial for the fasting lifestyle, because we don't want to lose lean muscle mass when we're fasting. We want our bodies to draw energy from their fat stores. Using your muscles and bones is a powerful way to give that signal to your body.

Basic Principles

Assuming you've got the diet side right, regular exercise completes the deal. Playing a hard game of basketball once a month and otherwise sitting in front of a screen is a bad routine. So is working out hard every day with no time for rest and recovery. If you can, try to work out four to six days a week. Focus on resistance training (RT) such as weight lifting, as well as High Intensity Interval Training (HIIT)—which I'll explain below.

If you have a busy week when you can only work out once or twice, then you can do full body workouts that combine all muscle groups. Just make sure your body has plenty of time to recover between these workouts (two to three days).

Reps (Repetitions) and Sets

In one workout, you want to do three to five different exercises per muscle or muscle group, for a total of nine to twelve sets. Within sets, shoot for six to twelve reps. One set is a series of reps with no rest in between. Don't spend more than an hour on an intense resistance workout unless you're an elite athlete.

Time-Under-Tension (TUT)

During a set, work to keep the muscle or muscle group under tension throughout the entire set. Your goal is not to move the weight. It's to exhaust a muscle or muscle group over most of its range of motion. Normally during a set, you don't want to lock out your joint, or allow a weight to hang or rest—unless you're training for complex callisthenic holds.

Move slowly enough so you can focus on the key muscle or muscle group.

Don't let it "rest" in the middle of a set. A set should last twenty to sixty seconds.

Muscle Groups to Work Out Together in Resistance Training (RT)

- **Chest** (pectorals), **triceps**, and **shoulders** (deltoids). You can also work out shoulders on a separate day. Note that these are mostly pushing muscles.
- **Back** (latissimus dorsi and trapezius) and **biceps**. Note that these are mostly pulling muscles.
- **Legs**, **butt** (glutes), **thighs** (quadriceps), **hamstrings**, **calves** (soleus and gastrocnemius), and **lower back**. You can work out calves more often than the large muscles above the knee. You can also add calf workouts to other days. Do lower back work at the *end* of the workout, since you need these muscles for strength and stability during other leg exercises.
- **Abs** and **obliques**: You can add these to any workout above, but never do them before you work out your legs. It's okay to do high repetition sets on abs. (Abdominal and core muscles are different from other muscles in your body.)

Don't spend too much total time on abs. You should get through an ab routine in fifteen minutes or less. They need far less rest between sets than other parts of your body.

Lift hard and then give your muscles time to recuperate.
Work out muscles and muscle groups hard enough to exhaust them, and then give them time to recover and rebuild. Don't do resistance training on the same muscles two days in a row.

Don't do hard RT on the same muscles more than three times per week. One to two times a week is plenty. And get lots of sleep.

Always warm up.

It's easy to injure muscles, joints, tendons, and ligaments in resistance training. *Always* take time to warm up muscles and joints *beforehand* and stretch the muscles *after* the workout.

Push the envelope.

It's a bad use of time to do resistance training with weight so light that you can easily do fifteen or more reps before failing. Shoot for roughly six to twelve reps on every set. The weight should be heavy enough that you can't do even one more rep. Normally, rest for thirty to sixty seconds between sets.

If you can do more than twelve reps in a set, increase the weight. If you reach a plateau where you simply can't go heavier at six reps, then it's time to change your routine.

Don't believe the myth that lifting heavy weight will cause you to "bulk up." It won't. Women rarely have that problem unless they're taking steroids and growth hormone.

Mix it up.

Don't do the same workout over and over. Your body will adapt to the same routine within a few weeks. If your muscles are not sore the day after a workout, that means the muscles have adapted. It's time to change. You can vary the weight and number of reps, the types of exercise, and the order of exercises. You can alternate sets of different exercises, rather than doing all two or three sets of the same exercise in a row. You can move between muscle group exercises (such as squats) and isolation exercises (like leg extensions on a machine.)

You can rotate between different exercises and machines. You can do drop sets. That's when you do several sets in a row, with little rest in between, dropping the weight on each successive set. You can do supersets, where you move straight from a set of one exercise to a set of another exercise on the same muscle group with no rest in between. You can change the speed and time-under-tension of reps and sets, and you can change the amount of rest time between sets.

That's a lot of choice. To help you remember, think "FIT": frequency, intensity, and time.

Protein, Fat, and Not a Lot of Carbs

For muscles to recover from resistance training, you need enough digestible protein in your diet, probably between one half and one gram per pound of your ideal body weight per day.

Here's a simple policy: On non-keto days, still try to keep carbs below one hundred grams per day and go for those with a low glycemic load. If you're insulin sensitive and avoid sugars and high-glycemic carbs—except immediately after working out—you probably won't have to count calories.

Anaerobic and Aerobic Exercise

Resistance training builds lean muscle mass, strengthens your muscles and bones, and increases your metabolism (and hunger). But it's anaerobic exercise. It doesn't require you to keep your pulse rate high for a sustained period. For that, you need aerobic exercise. The most efficient form of aerobic exercise is HIIT: high intensity interval training. Check out the many (free) HIIT workouts at www.fitnessblender.com.

Long, slow aerobic exercise is easier, but it takes up more time and is not as useful as HIIT for overall fitness, unless you're training for a marathon or are in the middle of a long fast. That said, you should try to walk as much and as often as you can. We're designed to walk. Just don't pretend that a leisurely walk is the same as an aerobic workout.

Fasting from food doesn't mean you have to fast from exercise. On the contrary, on fast days, you should be able to work out just as you would on non-fasting days, at least once your body has adapted.

WEEK FOUR

Three Days with One Meal a Day (23/1)

L ast week, we narrowed our feeding window to just four hours of every day, but we didn't try to reduce net calories over the course of the week. This week, we'll amp things up a bit. You still won't try to reduce how much food you eat, though you may find that you'll eat less on fasting days than you normally would.

Strictly speaking, you'll still be fasting intermittently, but some days will differ from others. Some days will look like last week—a ketogenic diet and a limited window for eating. Other days will look far more like a fast. On those days, you eat all your food in a one-hour time window.

And as in previous weeks, you have one mini-feast day on Sunday.

The Warrior Diet

In 2002, a former member of the Israeli Special Forces, Ori Hofmekler, published a book called *The Warrior Diet*.[1] The diet, he argued, mimics the diet and training of ancient Greco-Roman soldiers. It also taps into a more primal and instinctual way of eating. Hofmekler promised to show would-be warriors how to gain muscle and energy, slay body fat and metabolic problems, and conquer hunger and cravings.

There have been a zillion versions of this diet since Hofmekler proposed it. But the basic idea is simple: You under-eat for most of the day—think little snacks of egg and veggies. Then you have one big omnivorous meal at night. Just like the Vikings did after a day of raiding Christian villages in Northumbria. Skoal!

Or not. Who knows? We really don't have much data on how such groups ate, since they didn't leave behind many cookbooks. Still, this was a clever marketing pitch to all those guys who spent more time playing video games, getting tattoos, and watching Viking documentaries than they did working out at the gym.

And it paid dividends. Almost anyone who switched from the standard American diet circa 2001 to the Warrior Diet would see good results in the short run. Then they'd take to the internet to spread the word.

23/1 Intermittent Fasting

Hofmekler published his book at the peak of the six-meals-a-day fad. That made his diet seem wild and transgressive. Looking back on it from the present, though, it looks a lot like intermittent fasting. It rejects the claim that we're better off grazing. Instead, it seeks to amplify the contrasting cycle between fasting and feasting during a single day.

The little meals he proposed early in the day make sense for people who are trying to eat this way every day. Without small snacks followed by a big meal, many people would under-eat. In that case, the Warrior Diet could end up as just a low-calorie diet with all the calories consumed at once. This might still be better than a low-calorie grazing diet. But, as we've noted, underfeeding for weeks or months on end slows down your metabolism.

At the same time, the little snacks blunt the effects of fasting to reduce blood sugar and insulin and boost ketones. So many people now do an updated version of the Warrior Diet. They fast from food for twenty-three hours of the day and then eat as much as they want (of keto-friendly foods) during one hour in the early evening.

Some folks, such as fitness blogger Edward Vasquez, follow this 23/1 intermittent fast every day. (It's also called the OMAD Diet—one meal a day.) Vasquez is a bodybuilder, and so is very careful to get all the calories he needs during that one long meal. To judge from his videos, he manages to maintain plenty of muscle and low body fat on this routine.[2]

The method also has a noble foundation in Christian history. In his Rule, St. Benedict prescribed one meal a day, and as a result, it became a common monastic practice for many centuries. It might seem hardcore now, but recall that St. Benedict's Rule was designed, in part, to *moderate* the extreme ascetic practices of some early Christian monks.

What to Do This Week

Don't worry. You won't go OMAD every day this week. We'll use it as one step to reach our summit: the fasting lifestyle. On days one, three, and five, you'll limit your eating window to one hour. In other words, you'll eat one big meal.

On days two, four, and six, you can eat what you need over

an eight- to ten-hour period. As before, try to stay in ketosis. Eat until you're satisfied—not stuffed. Then stop.

On your OMAD days, you will spend most of a twenty-four-hour day in a fasted state. As a result, it's a good idea to ease into your one big meal. Here are a few tips:

- Start the meal with a warm glass of chicken stock or, better yet, bone broth. Don't dig right into a T-bone fried in butter. Your stomach needs to warm up. It's been in fasting mode for hours.
- Don't force-feed. Eat over the course of the full hour.
- As before, you need to get at least three-fourths of your calories from natural fats, no more than 20 percent from proteins, and 5 percent or less from carbs. The carbs should come from vegetables, mostly green vegetables that grow above ground. For instance, spinach, bok choy, broccoli, lettuce, watercress, asparagus, cabbage, collard greens, cauliflower, Brussels sprouts, kale, zucchini, mushrooms, peppers, and cucumbers.
- Don't forget to drink *lots* of water all day and keep up your intake of electrolytes (sodium, magnesium, potassium).
- On days one, three, and five, when you eat only one meal, don't try to restrict calories. You can eat as much in your one meal as you would across a normal day. But you probably won't do that. If you're not eating sugar, starches, and simple carbs, then it's hard to eat three regular meals in one sitting. Trust me. I've tried it. You could try drinking little cups of oil, but I wouldn't advise that unless you want your meal to go right through you. Eat normally, and you may just manage to get in a regular day's worth of calories.

And as long as you pay attention to natural signals of satiety, you won't eat too much.

Mini-Feast

On day seven, have a mini-feast. Eat throughout the day but keep it within a twelve-hour feeding window. Add in some low-glycemic fruit, such as half of a red grapefruit or a handful of berries. Mix them with whipped cream, either unsweetened or with a bit of liquid stevia or Truvía. Have a dark chocolate fat bomb.

Fat Bomb Recipe

1 $8\frac{1}{2}$-ounce bar unsweetened chocolate

$\frac{1}{2}$ cup coconut oil

3 tablespoons unsweetened cocoa powder

$2\frac{1}{2}$ teaspoons Truvía or similar sweetener

$\frac{1}{2}$ teaspoon liquid stevia (we use Trader Joe's brand)

1 teaspoon salt

$2\frac{1}{2}$ cups unsweetened coconut flakes

Put the coconut flakes on a cookie sheet. Toast them at 325°F until brown and crispy. Melt the unsweetened chocolate bar and coconut oil in a double boiler. Swirl in cocoa powder, sweeteners, and salt, and toasted coconut flakes.

With a spoon, put the mixture in the compartments of a cupcake pan. (We use a twelve-cupcake pan and put in silicone holders to make it easy to remove the goodies.)

Place in freezer for about ten minutes to solidify, then store at room temperature.

Eat such treats on a full stomach and later in the day, so they have less impact on your blood sugar. If you've avoided sugars, simple carbs, and most artificial sweeteners for the last couple of weeks, these will taste *much* sweeter than you expect.

Remind Me. Why Am I Doing This?

Remember, you've spent most of your life running off of sugar. You've also trained your body, like a caged rat, to expect food at certain times of the day. Your gut-brain axis is gonna push that little button for food whether you plan to eat or not. Your tongue will feel sad and bored. Your belly will goad you to eat every few hours by sheer habit and to boost your blood sugar, which is used to spiking and dropping like a radio wave. All this makes fasting hard. You might be able to fast here and there, but only by sheer acts of the will. And you probably wouldn't ever get the real benefits of fasting since all of your effort would be channeled into keeping yourself away from the Chips Ahoy! in the pantry.

With the plan you're on right now, though, you're learning to resist these pests. You're shifting your body from sugar-burning to fat-burning. To do that, you need to keep insulin levels low and become far more insulin sensitive. Eating a ketogenic diet and spending a big chunk of some days in the fasting state will help speed that process along.

The good news? By the end of this fourth week, you will be far more adapted to fasting. You'll be on your way to metabolic flexibility. And you won't have had to endure a single day when you had to restrict calories.

Fasting to Clear Your Mind

The first benefit of fasting that I personally experienced was mental clarity. As I mentioned in chapter 6, it happened after I had been eating a low-carb diet and then embarked on a thirty-six-hour fast. About twenty-four hours in, my mind suddenly felt supercharged. It was like the sensation of "flow": Distractions fell away, and one thought followed easily from another.

I went to the internet to do some research. I soon found scads of testimonies from fasters and keto-diet fans who reported the same experience.

Why would depriving myself of food clear my mind? Even without knowing the details, this effect bespeaks good engineering. Assume you wanted to design the human metabolism for survival over the long haul of human history. Isn't this how you'd do it? After all, our brain is our most important survival organ. What if the brains of early humans slowed down and their thoughts scattered to the winds whenever they missed a meal or two—just when they most needed to hunt and forage for food? This trait would have gotten weeded out of the gene pool after a few centuries of erratic food supply. Since we're still here, we can assume that our ancestors enjoyed some metabolic way to survive the frequent bouts of scarcity. And we have inherited the same metabolic system, even if we rarely need to use it in the twenty-first century.

Most people who fast more than a couple of days get a glimpse of the clarity of mind that often results. And many accomplished fasters report feeling better when they're fasting. "Our human nature often asks for more than what it needs, and sometimes the devil helps so as to cause fear about the practice of penance and fasting," wrote St. Teresa of Ávila. "My health has been much better since I have ceased to look after my ease and comfort."[1]

But what causes this? Well, we know that when we enter into a fasted state, our body boosts the hormones that excite our sympathetic nervous system, which you've probably heard referred to as the fight-or-flight response. That alone would be enough to counteract feelings of weakness. But this can't be the whole story. I sometimes have a fight-or-flight response when I get my blood drawn or hear a loud noise. In the first case, my blood pressure drops. In the second, my pulse rate spikes. But neither of these sensations is anything like the lucidity that I often experience while fasting. As I write this, I'm thirty-nine-thousand feet in the air flying to Austin, Texas. I'm well into a twenty-three-hour fast, and a feeling of placid euphoria has just come over me. I assure you that it's not the flight.

Once I really shifted to the fasting lifestyle, and quit grazing on sugar, my mental function improved enough that it created a massive disincentive ever to go back. I now fast, if possible, before I have a stressful presentation, media interview, or debate. And I've written a lot of this book while fasting.

This mental clarity would likely happen to many people who just never reach the stage where they experience it. It only takes about two weeks to break a sugar addiction. But if you imagine misery for as far as the eye can see when you cut sugar from your diet, then you're not likely to try it even for two weeks.

We don't yet have the full story about how fasting boosts brain function, but we can piece together threads of evidence to form a working theory. One important thread is ketones themselves, which seem to be a high-octane brain fuel. Ketones, unlike regular fatty acids, can cross the blood-brain barrier. And ketosis, whether achieved by diet, fasting, or both, is certainly *associated* with mental clarity. Many people report that the sensation is really strong when blood ketone levels reach the threshold of "nutritional ketosis"—about one mmol/L (millimoles per liter). If you've managed to reach that threshold in the last few weeks, you may have experienced the mental boost already. If so, you don't need me to describe it to you.

Our brains are only about 2 percent of our body weight but consume about 20 percent of our energy. Ketosis solves the problem that most humans dealt with for most of history: hungry brains and an inconstant food supply. Our brains do just fine running on stored body fat. Ketosis also protects the brain from the roller coaster of the carb-glucose cycle. If you wanted humans to be able to survive gaps in food supply, this is just how you'd design them.

Ketosis may be more than just a backup system, though. The brain seems to like ketones. Ketosis boosts the mitochondrial density not just in our muscles and internal organs, but in our brain as well.[2] These power plants in our cells can get more energy per unit of ketones than they can get from glucose. They can also convert ketones to ATP (the cell's fuel) with fewer destructive free radicals than when converting glucose.[3] Ketones are a cleaner fuel for the brain.

Fasting has been shown specifically to increase the body's production of a growth hormone called BDNF—brain derived neurotropic hormone. One important study showed that just a few weeks of intermittent fasting boosted BDNF levels by 50 to 400 percent. Fasting also triggers the release of other protein chaperones that protect brain health.[4] All this allows us to repair damaged neurons—despite what you may have been told in elementary school about how our brains are fixed at birth, and only degrade after that.

Fasting also increases the "plasticity" and strengths of synapses, which are the tiny portals that connect neurons to each other.[5] Synapses are the channels by which chemical neurotransmitters are sent between our neurons, and which modulate our mood. We want our synapses to be flexible or "plastic" so that they can adjust our moods properly. When they're working optimally, we have more conscious control over our emotional state. A single neuron may connect, by way of synapses, to a hundred thousand other neurons!

Fasting has even been shown to lower the levels of neurotransmitters that signal anxiety and depression and raise the levels of those that signal calm and contentment. One study looked at twenty-nine fasters during the Muslim month of Ramadan. It found that over the month, the levels of BDNF, NGF (nerve growth factor), and serotonin went up, especially at the end of the fasting period.[6] (In Ramadan, you'll recall, Muslims do not eat or drink when the sun is up.) Low levels of serotonin are linked to depression, and this neurotransmitter also helps regulate our sleep, appetite, and sex drive.

What About Glucose?

Of course, your brain still needs some glucose, even if you are deep in ketosis. It can get about 75 percent of its energy from ketones, but it needs the rest to come from sugar. Does that mean you need to chug sugar or carbs to keep your brain working? Not at all. You don't *need* to consume any sugar, since your body has two work-arounds to create glucose even if none is coming in. Your liver can convert protein to glucose through gluconeogenesis. Or, if there is no protein around, it can take the glycerol from fat molecules and turn that into glucose.

So don't spend time worrying that when you fast, you'll starve your brain. If you're metabolically flexible and otherwise healthy, your brain will do just fine.

Your Second Brain

Did you know that hundreds of millions of neurons, that is, brain cells, line your *gut* from one end to the other? I did not learn this in my human biology course in college in the 1980s. That's because most of what we know about this enteric nervous system, often called the "gut-brain axis," is the fruit of research in the last two decades. We're just now starting to grasp the broad outlines of this surprising reality.

Researchers now suspect that the link between the brain in

your head (with its one hundred billion neurons) and your "second brain," your gut, is central to your health and your mood. These two "brains" are constantly communicating with each other through a direct line called the vagus nerve. Most of their transmissions are outside of our conscious control.

This realization gives scientific substance to something that we already sensed. We talk about having "gut reactions," not having the "stomach" for certain experiences, and feeling butterflies in our stomach. If you are trying to make a tough decision and the reasons for each choice are equal, a friend may ask: "What does your gut tell you?" In other words, "What does your pre-rational instinct incline you to do?" This is an old idea. In the Old Testament, the Hebrew often locates deep emotions, not in the head or even the heart, but in the bowels. This detail tends to be lost in English translations.

We know from both animal and human studies that some kinds of emotional stress can mess with the signals sent between the two brains and cause gastrointestinal problems. And it works the other way too. G/I problems can lead to emotional distress.

Microbiome

This information superhighway between brain and gut does not just transmit messages from one part of the body to the other. Its southern end is crowded with trillions of bacteria and other microscopic creatures that occupy different parts of your gut. We call them the "microbiome." You may have a thousand species living inside you. There are more microbial cells *in* your body than there are cells *of* your body. These little messengers send all sorts of signals and play a role in our mood, our immune system and health, and our food cravings.

In fact, our gut bacteria produce much of the serotonin that our brains need in order to function. Fecal transplant experiments with mice have been shown to cure obesity and metabolic syndrome,[7] which are diseases not just of digestion but also of hormones and neuroregulation. Fifty years ago, most nutrition researchers would have laughed at the suggestion that putting healthy poop in the gut of a sick mouse could cure it. Today, the National Institutes of Health maintains a Human Microbiome Project.[8] How many other secrets of the brain-gut axis are still waiting to be discovered?

Where the Good Guys Come From

Gut health is all about helping the good guys protect us from the bad guys. But where do the good guys, called probiotics, come from in the first place? Your microbiome is a complex result of your birth, your upbringing, your environment, your emotional state, and your diet. Probiotic supplements have become popular in recent years as consumers have heard rumors of their benefits. But we still don't know exactly what proportion is ideal, or even if different people do better with different probiotics.

Whatever the benefits of supplements, they have not been our source of probiotics for most of our history. Instead, pretty much every traditional cuisine included fermented foods teeming with good bacteria. You should follow tradition here if you want to promote the health of the ecosystem in your G/I tract. Sauerkraut, kimchi, pickles, tofu, kombucha, unfiltered apple cider vinegar, yogurt, and kefir are all good sources (though watch the sugar with yogurt and kefir products). Just make sure you get the stuff that is really fermented. Some pickled vegetables and most tofu are merely soaked in brine and/or vinegar and don't contain the live bacteria you want.

Feeding Your Microbiome

Like all other forms of life, your gut microbiome needs fuel— called *pre*biotics—which it gets from your diet. Think of *pro*biotics as the seeds in your garden. The fuel is the soil and fertilizer. Depending on the soil and fertilizer we supply, we can end up with either a bumper crop or a weed-infested field. Our diet should encourage the presence of good bugs and drive away the bad. On the bad side: Too much sugar can encourage the fungus *Candida*, crowding the good guys out of precious real estate. This, in turn, can lead to fatigue, weight gain, bloating, irritable bowel syndrome, and constipation. And if you're feeding the sugar-lovers in your gut, you should expect them to send signals to your brain that you will encounter as sugar cravings. You probably already realize that, even if sugar gives you a short-term boost, it's a bad way to sharpen your focus.

On the good side: if you get most of your carbs from green and leafy vegetables, you will favor different biota than if you eat lots of refined sugar and carbohydrates. You want your gut to be lined with neon signs that say: *Goodbye simple-sugar lovers, hello veggie lovers*. This starts with a choice to eat in a certain way. And if you keep at it, you'll start to receive positive feedback that encourages the choice.

I've experienced this directly. I don't recall ever craving vegetables when I got hungry until I radically changed my diet. I thought about corn chips, Cheez-Its, and cheeseburgers. After three or four months of both fasting and a ketogenic diet packed with veggies, however, I lost the sugar cravings and gained a strong craving for veggies. If I have gone all day without eating, or without vegetables, I will pine for a big salad. It's hard to know just what role my changing microbiota have played in this, but I suspect they're key players.

The good bacteria thrive on the soluble fiber in vegetables and other plants. We can't digest this fiber on our own, so it passes through our stomach and small intestines. When it reaches the large intestine, it should encounter bacteria that can ferment and consume it. We, in turn, benefit from the by-products of this process—which include not just happy-making brain chemicals but also nutrients that feed our intestinal wall, which in turn fends off substances that might otherwise end up in the bloodstream and make us sick or miserable.

Besides fermented foods and soluble fiber, other prebiotics include omega-3 fats, found in oily fish and in large amounts in your brain, and foods rich in polyphenols, such as green tea, coffee, cocoa, and olive oil.[9]

Does Fasting Help Your Microbiome?

There's evidence that fasting can help you maintain a healthy microbiome, though we don't yet know exactly why. One study with fruit flies found a link between intermittent fasting, longer life, and "long-lasting gut health."[10] Some researchers have speculated that long fasts may allow our gut to rest and recover. "Fasting is very similar to rebooting the hard drive in a computer," says Alan Goldhamer, an author of one such study.

"Sometimes, the computer gets corrupted, and you do not know exactly where the problem is. But if you just turn it off and reboot it, a lot of times, that corruption gets cleared out. We develop issues, and when you turn the system down with fasting and allow it to reboot, a lot of things—from gut flora and microbiota in the gut to chronic inflammatory conditions—tend to sort themselves out."[11]

For more on the subject of feeding, fasting, feasting, and brain health, check out *Genius Foods* by Max Lugavere and Paul Grewal, and *Brain Maker* by David Perlmutter.[12] If you have a healthy diet and a good fasting routine, your brain, and with it your mind, should be much better off.

Can We Mimic a Fast and Still Get the Benefits?

Several years ago, BBC Two approached Dr. Michael Mosley about doing a documentary on intermittent fasting. The documentary, *Eat, Fast, and Live Longer,* aired in the UK in 2012, and was a sensation in the British Isles. (You can now watch the whole thing free on YouTube.)

Before he starts his investigation, Mosley is skeptical but open-minded. In the film he surveys the mounting scientific evidence in favor of calorie restriction. He even interviews one of the estimated one hundred thousand "cronies" worldwide. These are people who "chronically restrict" (CR) their intake of calories in pursuit of health and long life. It's not starvation. We're talking a few hundred calories per day below normal. Still, it takes serious discipline, which is surely why only about seven in every five hundred thousand of the global population do it by choice!

When Mosley compares his own health markers with those of "crony" Joe, the contrast is stark. Both are in their mid-fifties and about the same height. But Joe has 11.5 percent body fat, while Mosley has more than twice that—27 percent.

And Mosley's fat is especially concentrated in his mid-section, where it causes far more problems than the fat just under the skin. (Recall that the fat that accumulates around your organs and your abdomen is called "visceral fat." The fat under your skin, called "subcutaneous fat," is less of a concern.)

Still, Mosley doesn't see himself restricting calories for the rest of his life. "I cannot in all honesty imagine doing what Joe does," he admits, "which creates something of a dilemma. So, what I really want to do is try to understand the *ways* in which calorie restriction works. Then hopefully I can get all the delicious benefits without actually having to do it."

This leads him to Dr. Valter Longo of the University of Southern California. Longo is the head of USC's Longevity Institute and has dedicated his life to research on how to prolong life. Longo shows Mosley mice genetically engineered to have very low levels of a growth hormone called insulin-like growth factor 1 (IGF-1). The mice are much smaller than their unmodified cousins, but they live about 40 percent longer. From his research, Longo has concluded that IGF-1 is a key reason that calorie restriction increases longevity.

More evidence for this comes from a very rare group of people who have a condition called Laron syndrome. (There are only some 350 such people in the world.) "The very low levels of IGF-1 their bodies produce means they are short," Mosley explains in a related article, "but this also seems to protect them against cancer and diabetes, two common age-related diseases."[1]

IGF-1 pushes our cells to divide, so we need it to grow. But when our body is in "go-go mode" all the time, it prevents the body's cells from undergoing maintenance. When this growth hormone is low, however, cells in the body go into a protective mode, when they start to repair. (More on this later.) The stem cells in particular turn on, and these help counteract damage from aging.

It's protein in our diet, Longo thinks, that keeps cells in go-go rather than repair mode. "It's like driving your car all the time, and never taking it to the mechanic," he tells Mosley as they cruise down a California highway in a vintage Ferrari. Something is bound to go wrong. Fortunately, Mosley explains, "You don't have to be a crony to lower IGF-1. There is another way: fasting." To see these regenerative benefits, Longo advises a fast of three and a half days—three days and four nights. He recommends people do this once a month until their test results get where they should be.

Mosley tries it, under Longo's supervision. He consumes nothing but water, tea, coffee, and one twenty-five-calorie cup of salty miso soup per day. This long fast goes about as you might expect. Mosley suffers sleepless nights, and dreams about food. Still, it pays off. His blood work shows that his IGF-1 levels have plummeted—to nearly half of where they were just four days earlier.

"The biggest problem with prolonged fasting is me," Mosley confesses. "I just can't bring myself to do it." So he looks for an alternative that will make fasting more "palatable."

That takes him to Chicago to meet Dr. Krista Varady, who does experiments with alternate-day fasting. This involves a regular "feed" day followed by a day when subjects eat only a fourth of their daily energy needs—four hundred to six hundred calories depending on one's size. Rather than a strict fast, every other day *mimics* a fast by allowing just a little eating.

After a bit more research on alternate-day fasting, Mosley

opts for what he calls a "less extreme" version: the 5/2 fasting-mimicking diet. He commits to try it for five weeks.

The protocol is simple: During five days of the week, you eat the normal amount. On two days, however, you eat a very-low-calorie diet, about one-fourth of your usual daily intake—around five hundred calories for the average person. (So, four hundred calories for a small woman, and six hundred for a large man.) This is much lower than the two-fifths cut in calories often advised on calorie-restricted diets, leaving 1,200–1,500 calories per day. The difference between fasting-mimicking and dieting is that you don't fast every day. As a result, your body responds differently than if you just tried to cut calories every day.

Mosley eats what he wants on regular feed days. Still, after just five weeks, his scores improve—a lot.

He has lost both weight and body fat, and his waist size is smaller. Body fat has dropped from over 27 percent at the beginning of his journey, to just under 20 percent at the end. His total cholesterol has gone down, and his "good" HDL, up. And his blood sugar has dropped from pre-diabetic levels down to the normal range.

Key for Mosley, though, is the drop in IGF-1 levels. The weekly 5/2 routine had the same effect as the longer fast he endured with Valter Longo. It cut his levels *in half*. This has implications not just for short-term health, but for longevity as well.

Although it's not mentioned in *Eat, Fast, and Live Longer*, which came out in 2012, Valter Longo doesn't work just with genetically engineered mice. He has also studied the effects of fasting on the little rodents as well. We've known since the 1930s that mice and rats live longer and healthier lives if they are put on a calorie-restricted diet. Of course, the diet only works because scientists can put them in cages and control what the poor critters eat down to the last pellet. But would you even want to live to be 110 if, to do so, you had to endure hunger every day of your long life? Count me out.

The good news is that Longo has found that putting mice on a fasting-mimicking diet has many of the same perks as persistent calorie restriction. Indeed, the diet boosted the median life spans of mice in control groups by 11 percent.[2] That's just the median. Some calorie-restricted mice live a lot longer than that. Mice are good study subjects, since they are mammals like we are, but with much shorter life spans. That makes its feasible to do longevity studies on them.

There is also recent evidence of this effect in monkeys. So, what about humans? Longo has found in a hundred-person clinical trial that human subjects who adopt the fasting-mimicking diet for five days a month improve various metabolic factors that may lead to longer and healthier lives. These include factors we've discussed already: lower blood sugar, lower blood triglycerides, greater insulin sensitivity, reduced inflammatory markers, and the like.

The studies behind his protocol are solid,[3] and they fit with mounting evidence on the health benefits of fasting. However, Longo's arguments about a permanently low protein and near-vegan diet tend to be based on personal preference and epidemiological studies of large populations, which can't separate correlation from causation. Many of the health arguments for vegetarian and vegan diets fall apart on closer inspection.[4]

A permanently low-protein diet also conflicts with other health goals, such as increasing and maintaining muscle mass.

Perhaps we'll discover that there's a trade-off between living as long as you can and boosting muscle mass—at least for some people. Maybe there's a trade-off between being a great athlete and living as long as possible. Do tiny people on low-protein diets have, on average, a better chance of living to be 110? Could be. But the evidence for this at the moment is circumstantial at best. What's more, in his 2018 book, Longo manages to combine solid clinical studies with all manner of speculation and dietary conventional wisdom—some of which is wrong.

Finally, the fasting-mimicking method he proposes—which lasts for five days once a month—is too complex for most folks to follow. I live and breathe this stuff, and I have a hard time figuring out how to comply with the fast. The cynic may argue that it's complex by design, since that creates a market for Longo's expensive line of dietary products—which will run you about $150 a week. I'm not a cynic about that, especially since Longo donates his proceeds to charity. Still: this is quite a hurdle for most people who want to fast long term.

In any case, for our purposes, the key lesson is this: you may get most of the health benefits from a multi-day fast if, on your fast days, you *cut your intake of calories by about 75 percent and keep protein low.* That's huge. In week five, we'll test it out.

WEEK FIVE

18

The 4/3 Fasting-Mimicking Diet

Two weeks ago, we introduced time-restricted eating or intermittent fasting. If you've kept up, then last week you did three non-consecutive twenty-three-hour fasts with one big meal near the end of the day. Perhaps you've never gone twenty-three hours without eating anything in your entire life. But if you're following our plan, I bet these fasts were a lot easier than you would have guessed when you started.

You've also had one mini-feast day per week—and may have enjoyed them more than giant feasts you've had in the past.

This week, we'll follow the lead of Michael Mosley. Our routine is a hybrid of the 5/2 diet and the alternating-day fast, which we can call the 4/3 fasting-mimicking diet. This is the first week when you'll need to keep an eye on your calories. On each of your three, non-consecutive fasting days, you should eat no more than four hundred to six hundred calories—depending on your size.

Like last week, pick three non-consecutive fast days, such as Monday, Wednesday, and Friday. On these days, you'll fast from food for twenty-three hours of the day and then eat only a small amount of keto-friendly foods during one hour later in the day. This isn't quite a full day fast. It's a fasting-mimicking diet combined with the alternate-day, one-meal-a-day routine that we introduced last week. Both of these methods have been developed for scientific reasons. But as we'll discover, they fit nicely with some common fasts in Christian history.

What should you eat on fast days? To keep protein low and the details simple, you can just eat two avocados with salt and lime juice (a little less if you're on the small side). You can eat the slices or make guacamole with them. We add a lot of fresh garlic and some pico de gallo. Avocados are high in fat, and almost all their carbs are fiber, so they do a nice job of filling your stomach and feeding your healthy gut bacteria. If you go this route, you'll be eating a vegan diet on fast days.

Another option: Take bone broth, which is mostly protein and gelatin, and boil it with lots of cabbage, celery, and spices. You might also try bone broth with collard greens, but be sure to boil the greens until they're soft. Pressure cooking them (especially with an Instant Pot) is the fastest way to do this. You can add some chicken, Italian sausage, and homemade meatballs (without filler); just don't overdo it. You need to keep calories and protein down. This option does a good job of filling up your otherwise empty stomach.

On days when I do a fasting-mimicking diet, I often combine the two options above. I eat guacamole made with one avocado; some cucumber slices; and a few bowls of the bone broth veggie soup. Not quite vegan, but pretty close.

It's great news to learn that we can get many of the health benefits of a longer fast while still eating a little bit during the day. This is not only easier for most people. It also matches many of the traditional fast days in Christian history—which allowed only a little low-protein food. And it fits nicely with the many fast days of Eastern Rite and Orthodox Lent that continue to this day.

Do you have to eat all of your food in one sitting? No. Michael Mosley often eats two tiny meals on his fast days, one in the morning and one in the evening, for a combined total of no more than six hundred calories. This might be okay long term. But right now, while you're trying to adapt to fasting, stick with one small meal if you can. It will allow you to experience a more traditional fast day—rather than the ersatz fasts most folks keep nowadays.

Fasting-mimicking doesn't offer any benefits over straight fasting. If anything, mimicking a fast mutes some of the perks of a full fast. So why do it? Simple. For most non-fasters, it's far easier to mimic an all-day fast than to fast all day, so they're more likely to succeed. Our goal is for you to make fasting part of your permanent lifestyle. If you can't manage to keep a fast for a single day, you'll never make it a habit. That's why you'll try mimicking an all-day fast before taking the longer leap.

The Non-Fasting Days

Don't follow Mosley's lead on non-fasting days. Remember, you're still getting acclimated to fasting. Don't drink a big glass of orange juice or eat refined white bread or a donut. That will make your life much harder on fast days. During days two, four, and six, in other words, eat just like you did last week. Eat the keto-friendly foods you need in the right proportion over an eight-to-ten-hour period. Stick with plenty of natural fats, moderate amounts of protein, and mostly leafy green vegetables for your carbs. Some full fat dairy such as heavy cream and hard cheese are also fine, as are nuts such as macadamia nuts, almonds, pecans, pistachios, pumpkin seeds, sunflower seeds, and walnuts. But don't blow past fifty grams of total carbs for the day—or whatever threshold you need to stay in ketosis.

As before, eat until you're satisfied—not stuffed. Then stop.

Mini-Feast

On Sunday, have another mini-feast. Eat throughout the (twelve-hour) day. Perhaps have a small sweet potato with a big dollop of butter, a glass of dry wine, or a handful of corn chips. Finish off dinner with some low-glycemic fruit, such as half of a red grapefruit, a handful of berries, a slice of watermelon, or a small apple. You might have a few pieces of very dark chocolate. If you like treats with artificial sweeteners, this is the day to indulge.

Remember, this is a *mini*-feast. These treats are options. Just choose one or two.

Also, eat such treats on a full stomach, so they will have less impact on your blood glucose and insulin. You're still adapting to fat burning, so you don't want to kick yourself out of that mode too soon.

As before, drink *lots* of water every day and keep up your intake of electrolytes (sodium, magnesium, potassium).

By the end of this week, you'll have what it takes to benefit from all-day fasts—and longer.

Fasting for Spiritual Warfare

It is impossible to engage in spiritual conflict, without the previous subjugation of the appetite.

—St. Gregory the Great

Remember Jesus's comment from the gospels that certain demons can only be driven out with prayer and fasting? In Matthew 17:21, for instance, Jesus, referring to an especially dug-in nest of demons, tells his disciples, "But this kind never comes out except by prayer and fasting." Did you know that this verse doesn't appear in many Bible translations? If you read the Revised Standard Version, as I do, you might notice that the text just skips from verse 20 to verse 22. In the King James Version, the verse is moved to a footnote. What's going on?

It turns out some ancient manuscripts include this verse, but the earliest ones do not.[1] When this type of text variant occurs among manuscripts, Bible scholars, including orthodox Catholic and evangelical ones,[2] tend to conclude that the text is a gloss that's been added later. Most scholars treat the verse in Matthew as an "interpolation" from Mark 9:29, which says, "This kind cannot be driven out by anything but prayer and fasting." As Michael Pakaluk observes, one of the key themes in Mark is that "a spiritual authority has arrived which can banish and subdue the devil."[3] (Though even in Mark, some ancient manuscripts mention only prayer and not fasting.)

No one can say for sure how to sort out the details, though for believing Christians, they don't really matter that much. The text is in the received canon, and we have no reason to assume Jesus didn't speak these words during his earthly ministry.

But let's assume, for the sake of argument, that this reference to prayer *and* fasting was added to Matthew by a scribe in the fifth century. Such scribes otherwise showed a fanatical commitment to preserving the ancient texts. So, why would one add a gloss about prayer and fasting? It helps to see the text that precedes it:

> *And when they came to the crowd, a man came up to him and kneeling before him said, "Lord, have mercy on my son, for he is an epileptic and he suffers terribly; for often he falls into the fire, and often into the water. And I brought him to your disciples, and they could not heal him." And Jesus answered, "O faithless and perverse generation, how long am I to be with you? How long am I to bear with you? Bring him here to me." And Jesus rebuked him, and the demon came out of him, and the boy was cured instantly. Then the disciples came to Jesus privately and said, "Why could we not cast it out?" He said to them, "Because of your little faith. For truly, I say to you, if you have faith as a grain of mustard seed, you will say to this mountain, 'Move from here to there,' and it will move; and nothing will be impossible to you."*

Think about this from the viewpoint of pious Christians living at the time. They were witnessing the principalities and powers of the Roman Empire being overthrown, by both the Visigoths and the Holy Spirit. Demon possession was a part of daily life, and a clear and present danger for Christians. Without the gloss, the text might give them the impression that only Jesus in the flesh, or a near-impossible faith, would drive out really powerful demons. For such Christians, that would be a counsel of despair. It might also have contradicted what they discovered through hard experience: fasting and prayer offer a supernatural power-up for doing spiritual battle, including even exorcisms. Under such circumstances, it makes sense why a scribe would want to add a line from the book of Mark to Matthew—as a reminder.

To this day, Canon Law requires priests to pray *and* fast ahead of time before performing an exorcism, and to admonish the victim of possession to do the same. St. Philip Neri once observed, "There is nothing the devil fears so much, or so much tries to hinder, as prayer." Perhaps early Christians, and the Church in her wisdom, found that there is one thing Satan fears even more: prayer and fasting. So, when you fast, do everything you can to pair it with prayer.

Preparing for Battle

Even without these texts, we have a great reason to connect fasting with spiritual warfare. After all, it's the stated purpose for the most dramatic fast in the New Testament: Jesus's fast of forty days and forty nights. Matthew, Mark, and Luke all report this event but are stingy with the details. Mark just mentions it in passing. Still, the texts provide hints for those with the eyes to see.

All three accounts agree, as Matthew writes, that Jesus "was led up by the Spirit into the wilderness to be tempted by the devil" (Matt. 4:1). What? Why would the Holy Spirit *want* Jesus to be tempted? Again, a little context helps clear things up. This event comes right after Jesus is baptized by John, and right before his public ministry, which would end in his violent death. His time in the desert, it seems, was like physical and spiritual basic training to fortify him for the onslaught to come. The Greek word for "tempt" in the text means something like "test" or "attempt." He was going to be taking on Satan and his many minions. This called for the mother of all boot camps.

And what did Jesus do? Hibernate in a cave? Lift weights? Carb load? Do high intensity interval training? Uh, no. "And he fasted forty days and forty nights," Matthew writes, "and afterward he was hungry" (Matt. 4:2). In light of what he did throughout his ministry, we can assume this was also a time of prayer.

Why forty? Why not thirty-nine or forty-one? Well, for some reason, forty has special meaning in God's plan of salvation. In the time of Noah, it rained for forty days and forty nights. Moses spent forty days and forty nights fasting on top of Mt. Sinai when he received the Ten Commandments from God. The Hebrews—God's chosen people—spent forty years in the desert after they left Egypt. Elijah fasted for forty days and forty nights during his long journey to Mt. Horeb (another name for Mt. Sinai).

In every case, the forty days/nights/years were a trial that came just before something new. God cleansed the earth of sin before starting a new covenant with Noah. The Hebrews' long sojourn in the desert was part punishment (for grumbling and building a golden calf) and part preparation before they entered the Promised Land. While in the desert, they had to depend day by day on water from rocks and on God's miraculous bread from heaven—manna—plus the occasional quail.

So, too, with Jesus in the desert. As Marcellino D'Ambrosio puts it, this was the prelude for "the birth of a new Israel liberated from sin, reconciled to God, and governed by the law of the Spirit rather than a law chiseled in stone."[4] The first Adam failed the test. The second Adam passed it.

Notice that it also takes about forty days to become keto-adapted after decades of using sugar for energy. Maybe that's just a coincidence. Or maybe not.

Don't Explain It Away

It might be tempting to explain away the whole episode. *Well, sure*, you might think. *Jesus is the Son of God. He can multiply fish and loaves of bread. I'm a mere mortal who could no more fast for forty days than I could raise up a guy who's been dead in the tomb for four days.* That's what I vaguely thought for a long time. It didn't occur to me that what Jesus did is, in some ways, a model for us as well. Note that the gospel writers go out of their way to tell us that Jesus *didn't* use miracles to get through the fast.

As Luke writes, "And he ate nothing in those days; and when they were ended, he was hungry" (Luke 4:2). That's the primary meaning of a fast. Fasting means *not eating*.

Then, after the fast, "the tempter came and said to him, 'If you are the Son of God, command these stones to become loaves of bread'" (Matt. 4:2). Satan's taunt to make bread from stones only makes sense if Jesus was feeling the hunger of his all-too-human body.

Notice also that Satan appealed to Jesus's hunger, but not to his thirst. We can assume that Jesus drank water because, without a miracle, no one could survive without water for forty days and nights.[5] (The angels did minister to Jesus, but only after his long fast and triple-testing from Satan.) But, believe it or not, a healthy person *can* fast from food for forty days. He just needs enough energy stored as fat on his body. There are 3,500 calories in a pound of fat. So thirty pounds of extra fat would be enough—not all that much for a well-fed man—as long as his body was able to access its fat stores.

What's This Got to Do with Me?

This doesn't mean you should do a forty-day, water-only fast, even if you could do so—with careful practice and planning. Jesus's forty-day fast in the gospels is a big, flashing neon sign to remind us that fasting should never have ceased to be a basic part of the Christian life. We miss part of what God intends for us if we try to explain it away.

Jesus's example helps put shorter fasts in perspective. It also gives us one of the best reasons to fast: to prepare for spiritual battle. If it's good enough for Jesus, it should be good enough for us.

This, by the way, is why hundreds of millions of Christians set aside forty days leading up to Easter, as a special time of preparation, fasting, and prayer.

Here's how Pope Benedict XVI describes Lent:

Lent is like a long "retreat" in which to re-enter oneself and listen to God's voice in order to overcome the temptations of the Evil One and to find the truth of our existence.

It is a time, we may say, of spiritual "training" in order to live alongside Jesus not with pride and presumption but rather by using the weapons of faith: namely prayer, listening to the Word of God and penance.

In this way we shall succeed in celebrating Easter in truth, ready to renew our baptismal promises.[6]

Don't forget that when you fast, you should take time to pray against evil spiritual strongholds in yourself, your family, your ancestry, your church, your country, and the world.

Don't know where to start? Commit the Prayer to St. Michael to memory and pray it throughout your fast. It only takes about fifteen seconds!

Saint Michael the Archangel,
defend us in battle,
be our protection against the wickedness and snares of the devil;
may God rebuke him, we humbly pray;
and do thou, O Prince of the heavenly host,
by the power of God, cast into hell
Satan and all the evil spirits
who prowl about the world seeking the ruin of souls.
Amen.

Michael, recall, is the archangel who defends Israel against the principalities of Persia in the book of Daniel. (He also makes an appearance in the New Testament, in Jude and Revelation.)

In both places, we find him fighting Satan and other demons. Pope Leo XIII wrote this prayer in the 1880s, reportedly after receiving a vision of demons descending on Rome.[7] He asked Catholics to pray this and a few other "Leonine" prayers at the end of every Mass. The practice continued through the 1960s, when it began to disappear. Many thought talking about Satan and demons was so out-of-date, so . . . medieval. Our twenty-first-century trials and tribulations—both outside and inside the Church—have led many priests and bishops to reinstitute this corporate prayer.

It's also a powerful private prayer. In fact, many priests use it during exorcisms and commend it to the faithful for fighting the devil. The prayer shouldn't be the only weapon in your private arsenal. But you should carry it with you, especially on fast days, like a spiritual stiletto.

20

Fasting to Lose Weight and Fight Diabesity

Can fasting cure obesity? That is, if you suffer from obesity and you stop eating, will you lose weight?

Of course you will. Consider the Scottish man Angus Barbieri, who in the mid-1960s fasted for 382 days. He subsisted on water, tea, coffee, vitamins, potassium, and sodium supplements until the very end of the fast.

Fasting for over a year wasn't his original plan. He just knew he had to do something. By the time he reached his twenty-seventh birthday, he had reached a corpulent 456 pounds with no end in sight. So he went to a clinic in Dundee to ask for help, and doctors there put him on a short fast. (Fasting was not considered a crazy idea in Scotland at the time.) Barbieri went home and stopped eating.

The doctors had advised him to fast for only a few days, to kick-start his weight loss. But to everyone's surprise, Barbieri kept at it. He had set a target of getting down to 180 pounds—far less than half his starting weight. That distant goal must really have motivated him, since his few days of fasting turned into weeks, and the weeks turned into months, and the months turned into a year, and then some. He did not stay in the hospital, though he returned to the clinic frequently for check-ups. Throughout the fast, he reported feeling fine. After the first few days, he didn't even feel hungry. By the end, he claimed to have forgotten the taste of some foods. After more than a year without food, he reached his goal of 180 pounds. Even years later, he had inched up only to 196 pounds.[1]

How did this work? Well, his body used his stored fat for fuel, *which is what it was designed to do.* Barbieri was obese because his metabolism had gone haywire years before. When you're eating the kind of food you're designed to eat, and your metabolism is working as it should, things don't get out of whack. You don't overeat or under-eat. In fact, some famous "overfeeding" experiments at the University of Vermont showed that healthy adults find it hard to overeat over the long haul. Force-feeding subjects caused weight gain at first. But then their weight leveled off. Why? Well, when you stuff your stomach with food, various hormones like leptin signal satiety, making it really tough to keep shoving food down your gullet. Some of the Vermont subjects disliked it so much that they dropped out on the study.

The extra calories also led subjects to burn more calories. "Total energy expenditure in the subjects increased by 50 percent," notes Jason Fung.[2] The rule seems to be, *Eat more, burn more.*

So how does a man like Angus Barbieri swell to 456 pounds? Only after spending years in a metabolic vicious cycle, eating foods that scramble natural hormonal signals. That's the claim of the hormonal theory of obesity, and there's far more evidence for it than there ever was for the cartoon version of the caloric theory we all take for granted.

In the extreme situation in which Barbieri found himself, an extreme dietary intervention fixed the problem.

I'm *not* suggesting that you follow his plan, even if you weigh 456 pounds. Barbieri embarked on a year-long fast with no short fasts to prepare his body. This is probably the riskiest fast imaginable. And afterward, one would risk something called "refeeding syndrome." Angus Barbieri is famous because he's the reigning world champion for long-term fasting. There are only a few other people known to have lived over 300 days without food. He's an outlier, not a model.

You should not be surprised that he lost body fat during the fast—it would a miracle if he didn't. What should surprise you is that he managed to keep the weight off. This surprised me. I would have expected that his basal metabolic rate would have ground to a halt and that he would have depleted his lean body mass. But he was in fine health afterward. If his metabolism slowed down, it must have just downshifted to the metabolism of a much smaller and leaner man. Unlike almost every contestant who has appeared on *The Biggest Loser*, Barbieri didn't regain all his old weight.

Happily for the obese, we now know there are much less severe ways to achieve the same result.

If you are severely overweight, fasting might be just the ticket to help you lose those extra pounds of blubber and keep them off. By this point, you know why. It will give you a sustainable way to take more control over your diet. And it will make you *metabolically flexible*, so that your body can use body fat as fuel, rather than storing it for a rainy day that never comes.

HOW TO DETERMINE IF YOU'RE OVERWEIGHT

Different people have different ideal weights. If you're really overweight, though, you know it already, even if you don't know the medical definition. There's no thick black line that distinguishes obesity from overweight, but there are official ways to measure where you are on the spectrum.

The first is your body-mass index (BMI). This is a ratio of your height to your weight. Here's the formula: $W/H^2 \times 703$, that is, weight (in pounds) divided by height (in inches) squared, multiplied by 703. That's hard to remember, but you can Google "bmi calculator" and one will come up. You just type in your weight and height, and it will give you your score.

THE BMI CATEGORIES ARE AS FOLLOWS:
    Underweight: less than 18.5
    Normal weight: 18.5–24.9
    Overweight: 25–29.9
    Obesity: 30 or greater
    Severe obesity: 35.0–39.9
    Morbid obesity: above 40

The key virtue of the BMI? It's easy to calculate. You just measure your weight and height and do a little arithmetic. But it has some vices as well. For one thing, it doesn't measure body fat, which is what matters. When we worry about being "overweight," we're not worried about muscle and bone weight. We're worried about too much body fat. The BMI is blind to the difference. A fit, muscle-bound person could register as overweight or even obese.

Take Arnold Schwarzenegger. At his peak, when he won several Mr. Olympia contests, he was 6'2" and weighed

235 pounds during competitions. So his BMI was 30.2, which ranked him as obese, even though he had less than 5 percent body fat! (For comparison, the average competitive marathon runner has around 10 percent body fat.)

If you're not a professional bodybuilder, though, the BMI is a decent first approximation.

The ideal is to measure body fat percentage. Very roughly, a healthy body fat percentage for most men will fall between 10 percent and 17 percent. (Even elite athletes rarely go below 10 percent.) For women, 21 to 24 percent is considered the normal healthy range, though very fit women may get down to 14 percent.

Notice that it can be unhealthy to be outside the range *on either end*. Extremely low body fat is a serious problem, especially for women—though it's not all that common. Competitive bodybuilders can bring their body fat down into the single digits, but only during competition. At the other end of the spectrum, anything above 26 percent for men and 31 percent for women is defined as obese.

There are several ways to measure body fat directly. The virtue of the methods is that they target what we really want to know. Their vices are cost and complexity. And the more accurate the method, the more complicated and expensive it is.

Fortunately, there's a third method for determining if you have too much of the (wrong kind) of body fat. It's free and easy. You just divide your waist circumference by your height in inches. Your waist should be no more than half your height. If your score is below 0.5, in other words, you're in pretty good shape. If it's above that, then you should lose some body fat for the sake of your long-term health.

Even simple time-restricted eating can make a big difference. A recent major study in *Cell* reported that subjects who restricted their eating window lost weight, even though they didn't change their diet or cut calories.[3] This suggests that the obesity epidemic is in part the result of most folks eating too often throughout the day, and never taking a real break from the fed state.

Of course, if you suffer from full-blown type 2 diabetes, this may be just the first step in reversing the disease.

Diabetes

Obesity isn't merely an aesthetic problem. It's harmful to our health, especially because of its association with type 2 diabetes. This disease tends to develop only after years of high blood sugar, so the link between it and diet might not be obvious at first.

There have been cases of obesity and type 2 diabetes throughout history. But they have reached epidemic numbers in the last few decades, especially in the US. "According to the Centers for Disease Control and Prevention," notes a heart-breaking essay in the *Huffington Post*, "nearly 80 percent of adults and about one-third of children now meet the clinical definition of overweight or obese. More Americans live with 'extreme obesity' than with breast cancer, Parkinson's, Alzheimer's and HIV put together."[4]

Almost 70 percent of the US army are overweight or obese![5]

And the disease is spreading to other countries as they adopt ever more features of the standard American diet. China, which for decades had low rates of diabetes, now looks like it's trying to catch up.

Obesity and type 2 diabetes are such common traveling companions that many researchers refer to them as a single condition, diabesity. Along the path from overweight to diabetes, one can start showing markers of bad health that researchers often refer to as "metabolic syndrome." This includes high blood triglycerides, low HDL ("good") cholesterol, high blood pressure, and high fasting blood glucose.

In his books *The Obesity Code* and *The Diabetes Code*, Jason Fung connects the dots. He describes in lucid detail how too much sugar can lead, over time, to both obesity and diabetes. Together, these two books present what may be the clearest and most persuasive case in print for the hormonal-imbalance theory of obesity.

Type 2 diabetes is so deadly because it leads to many other diseases. In fact, diabetes is a leading cause of heart attacks, strokes, cancer, kidney disease, blindness, nerve damage, and damage to extremities that lead to amputation. That's because, over time, it attacks every organ of your body.

Unfortunately, medicine often treats the symptoms of type 2 diabetes rather than its underlying cause. This started out innocently. Until the discovery of insulin by three scientists at the University of Toronto in 1921, type 1 diabetes was almost always fatal. A year after insulin was discovered, though, it was first used on patients with great success. It has since saved and lengthened the lives of millions of people.

With type 1 diabetes, the body attacks the beta cells in the pancreas that produce insulin. This causes them to fail, leaving the person with little or no insulin. People with this disease wither away because their bodies can't use the food energy they consume. The sugar they need for fuel gets filtered by the kidneys and passes out of the body during urination. Insulin injections restore the body's signaling system, so that it can use food for energy and store extra energy as fat.

Type 2 diabetes, in contrast, is not brought about by a lack of insulin—at least not at first—but rather from severe insulin-resistance brought on by *too much insulin*. Under the constant threat of invasion from sugar, the cells start to resist. This can go on for years, with the pancreas pumping ever more insulin into the blood to clear it of rising blood sugar levels. What can't be cleared returns to the liver, which converts the sugar to fat. That fat builds up around the internal organs, including the liver, which gets sluggish as a result, and the pancreas, which may start to lag behind in delivering enough insulin to do the job. As a result, blood sugar rises to dangerous levels and, if left untreated, ravages the body.

At this point, a doctor may start giving a patient insulin to treat the high blood sugar. The patient likely already has high insulin levels, but they're not high enough to clear the sugar from her bloodstream. Injecting insulin doesn't fix insulin resistance. It makes it worse.

Resistance is a natural response when the body is exposed regularly, over and over, to a substance. If you keep taking morphine, marijuana, cocaine, or alcohol without a break, your body will build up resistance to it. As a result, you'll have to take ever larger doses to produce the same effect. The same thing happens with insulin. At first, just a small dose may be enough to get a patient's blood sugar down into the normal range. But over time, he'll need larger and larger doses to get the same result. That means he'll have a consistently high insulin level, which is a surefire way to make someone fat.

As Jason Fung puts it in *The Obesity Code*:

> *I can make you fat.*
>
> *Actually, I can make anybody fat. How? By prescribing insulin. It won't matter that you have willpower, or that you exercise. It won't matter what you choose to eat. You will get fat. It's simply a matter of enough insulin and enough time.*[6]

The real villain is not the fat just under your skin, but the visceral fat that collects around your internal organs. This, in turn, feeds the diabetes in a deadly, vicious cycle.

But what if, for many diabetics, there's a drug-free alternative?

The work of Fung and others suggests that there is. They're helping patients control and even reverse type 2 diabetes through diet. Many are able to get off of insulin entirely. Can you guess what the diet involves? Yep: fasting, cutting out sugars and refined carbohydrates, and adding healthy natural fats. Surprised?

In severe cases, Fung may put diabetic patients on a seven- or even fourteen-day water-only fast. This serves to bring their blood sugar and insulin levels way down, that is, to reverse the process that made them diabetic in the first place.[7] Many of them end up on longer routines of twenty-four to thirty-six-hour fasts, two to three times per week. The results are impressive. The routines allow the body to establish a new, lower set weight (BSW), where it remains—as long as the patient doesn't return to old, bad ways of eating.

Their work is in its infancy, and more research needs to be done. It would be nice to have large, double-blind clinical trials to back it up. Still, the early results are inspiring. I predict that future studies will confirm the value of this protocol.

If you suffer from pre-diabetes or type 2 diabetes and want to find a drug-free way to fight back, you probably won't want to wait for clinical trials. Nor should you. Still, don't jump the gun—especially if you are on drugs to lower your blood sugar. *You need to be under a doctor's care before trying this yourself.* When you start fasting and eating a ketogenic diet, your blood sugar will drop. Injecting insulin, in particular, could then bring it down into the danger zone. You'll need to adjust your dose to keep that from happening. This is not something you should try at home without medical supervision.

I'd encourage you to read about the Intensive Dietary Management Program that Fung and Megan Ramos run in Toronto. You can get a lot of free information at their website: www.idm program.com. You can even set up a consulting appointment with them online without leaving your house. But you'll still need a local doctor to help you navigate the treacherous waters. Just be sure to find a doctor who isn't so skeptical of the plan in principle that he or she will try to talk you out of it.

A recent study with type 2 diabetics in *Metabolism* showed that over a twenty-four-hour period, fasting lowered subjects' blood sugar, insulin, and glucagon—a related hormone that tells the liver to convert stored glycogen into glucose. Fasting does this far more than a standard diet, and even more than a full-calorie, very-low-carb diet.[8] If you want to get these numbers down without drugs, there may be no more powerful tool in your arsenal than fasting.

The fasting lifestyle may help prevent and even reverse many diseases, some of which we'll discuss later. But it probably holds the most promise for reversing diabesity, since it targets the root cause of the disease. Heck, if this were the only health benefit of fasting, it would still be revolutionary, since it could halt a global epidemic.[9]

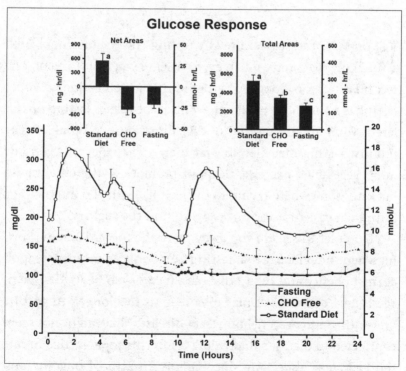

Nutall F. et al., *Metabolism* 64, no. 2: 253–62, "Comparison of a Carbohydrate-Free Diet vs. Fasting on Plasma Glucose, Insulin and Glucagon in Type 2 Diabetes."

21

Fasting to Fight Disease
and Live Longer

If you search "diseases cured by fasting" on the internet, you'll find cures for pretty much every disease you can think of. The second article on Google when I did this search is titled "Proper fasting is a cure-it-all medicine." This hype makes fasting no different from any other kind of diet intervention. Whatever the promise—a high-fat diet, low-fat diet, apple cider vinegar, raw milk, vegetables, exercise, sleep, or probiotics—there's always a huckster somewhere trying to oversell it. With the internet, it's just much easier for the hucksters to find the suckers.

Don't let this scare you away from the topic. There *is* growing scientific evidence that fasting is not only a powerful weapon against obesity and type 2 diabetes, it can even be used to manage type 1 diabetes.[1] It may also help us live longer, in part by preventing and even helping treat diseases that might not seem connected to diet. It's impossible to do this topic justice in one short chapter, especially since this is an area of ongoing and sorely needed research. Right now, we have more questions than answers. Still, let's summarize what we know so far.

Discordance

We already have good reason to suspect that the standard American diet and lifestyle play a role in the "diseases of civilization" or "Western degenerative diseases." Cultures with traditional diets were (and a few still are) largely free of such diseases, even among their elderly—it's not just that they all die too soon to get cancer or diabetes. Those that survive war and infectious diseases tend to have a "compressed mortality curve." That means they live a long, healthy life and then die quickly. Short of immortality, that's just what most of us would like to have.

So, what's the problem with our modern diet? It's not merely macronutrients. Different traditional diets vary radically in this way. Some are higher in fat, some higher in protein, some higher in carbohydrates. These different diets seem to cause different genes to be expressed to adjust to the respective diets. Traditional cultures with high-carb cuisines, for instance, tend to have more expression of amylase genes. (Amylase is the enzyme needed to digest starch.) Other cultures with extremely high-fat diets, such as the Greenland Inuit, may have genetic adaptations to their diets as well.[2]

Yet despite this variety, *none* of these diets includes large amounts of sugar, highly processed carbs, or industrial seed oils. It doesn't follow that these are the *cause* of every one of these maladies. Still, as we've seen, the evidence for the link between diet and disease grows daily. And the "discordance hypothesis" is a plausible way to explain these findings. "This mismatch between our ancient physiology and the western diet and lifestyle underlies many so-called diseases of civilization," argues one group of researchers, "including coronary heart disease, obesity, hypertension, type 2 diabetes, epithelial cell cancers, autoimmune disease, and osteoporosis, which are rare or virtually absent in hunter–gatherers and other non-westernized populations."[3]

One Friend's Testimony

While working on this book, I asked some friends if they'd be willing to test out the forty-six-day protocol and give me their feedback. My friend Anne gave me by far the most detailed reports. As soon as she switched to a ketogenic diet, she started losing a lot of weight. The dietary fats and mini-feasts made it far less challenging than she had imagined it would be. And once the intermittent fasting kicked in, other surprising things started to happen, which neither of us anticipated. Two months in, and her life had changed.

She sent this email to my wife and me (subject: "healing from fasting"):

> I have to share a testimony of what I think is God's heal-ing in my body: I was diagnosed with Polycystic Ovarian Syndrome (PCOS) when I was 18, at which point my insulin levels were already elevated to pre-diabetic, despite my (then) athletic lifestyle. The next 16 years brought weight gain and frustration, despite my efforts and medication. On Metformin or running half-marathons and training for more, my hormones were never under full control and my cycle was always very long and unpredictable. But in the last few months, with just a few 24- and 36-hour fasts, my cycle is finally in the normal range, which I never thought

I'd see, certainly not without medication. I haven't had my insulin checked in years, but my guess is that it's finally low enough to lower the testosterone and allow my body to function the way God designed it as a woman of child-bearing years. My mom and grandmother both probably had PCOS and certainly experienced diabesity and fertility issues, so I think it's safe to say that fasting (and prayer!) may have just reversed a hereditary disease in my body!

All of which to say, thank you so much for sharing this lifestyle with me; Jay, thank you for writing this book; and God bless us all to fast and be healed!

I've read scores of testimonies like this from others who have discovered the wonders of fasting. But it meant far more to me to get this news from a close friend. PCOS is just one of the diseases that can be treated with fasting.[4]

Alzheimer's

Near the end of his documentary *Eat, Fast, and Live Longer*, Michael Mosley travels to Baltimore to interview Dr. Mark Mattson. Mattson does research on Alzheimer's and fasting. Fasting, we learn, delays the onset of Alzheimer's in mice, compared to a fast-food diet—which includes fructose in their drinking water. What explains the difference? The researchers examined the mice who were fasting and found, as Mosley explains, that "sporadic bouts of hunger actually trigger new neurons to grow." Alternate-day fasting, Mattson says, "is better for the mouse brains than constant calorie restriction."

Some researchers are now calling Alzheimer's "type 3 diabetes," due to its perceived connection with diet.

There are several ways that fasting and ketosis may protect
the brain against degeneration—especially over the long term.
For instance, studies have found that the brains of Alzheimer's
victims seem to have trouble metabolizing glucose, while their
mental functions improve after several weeks of taking medium-
chain triglycerides. These are the fats found in abundance in
coconut oil—fats the liver easily converts to ketones. If you're
interested in strategies to prevent, or at least delay, the onset of
Alzheimer's, check out *The End of Alzheimer's* by Dr. Dale Bredesen and *The Alzheimer's Antidote* by nutritionist Amy Berger.[5]

Epilepsy and Parkinson's Disease

What about other neurological diseases? As far back as ancient
Greece, fasting was used to reduce the number of seizures in
children. In the twentieth century, a few doctors knew that a
ketogenic diet (which, like longer fasts, puts the body in ketosis)
could help treat childhood epilepsy. Unfortunately, official authorities dismissed this fact due to their bias against dietary fat.

Recent scientific research has confirmed the value of fasting
itself for this treatment. A 1999 paper from scientists at Johns
Hopkins explains their conclusion in the title: "Seizures decrease rapidly after fasting."[6] In the study, children were put on
a thirty-six-hour fast and then food "was gradually introduced
over three days." The benefit seemed to result from fasting-
induced ketosis, since other evidence suggests that a highly ketogenic diet alone may work.[7] If so, that's good news. Though
fasting jump-starts ketosis, most cultures have exempted small

children from the rigors of fasting. Still, there's evidence that the combination of diet and fasting improves outcomes.[8]

At the other end of life, Parkinson's disease also responds to ketosis. This disease degrades both mental and motor function. You may remember the growing weakness and trembling of Pope John Paul II, who suffered from Parkinson's during the final years of his life.

In one 2018 study, patients with Parkinson's who ate a ketogenic diet for eight weeks improved both their motor and non-motor skills (such as mental acuity).[9] Some researchers suspect that fasting, too, might help prevent, delay, and even treat the disease, though more research is needed.

Cancer

In the 1920s, German scientist (and future Nobel Laureate) Otto Warburg was studying cancer cells and made a startling discovery. He noticed that they draw almost all their energy anaerobically (without oxygen), by fermenting glucose (called glycolysis). One clue tipped him off: the cells produced lots of lactic acid, which is a by-product of glycolysis.

You need some background details to grasp why Warburg was surprised. You see, many organisms, from the simplest to the most complex, can derive energy in their cells in this way. But glycolysis is about eighteen times less efficient than aerobic metabolism, which requires oxygen. (Hence, aerobic metabolism is also called respiration.) That's why organisms use aerobic metabolism for most energy needs. Glycolysis tends to be used for short, intense energy needs when oxygen is not available. For humans, that might be lifting a heavy weight or running the hundred-meter dash. In a short sprint or heavy lift, your lungs and heart can't channel enough oxygen into the muscles to get the job done. That's when the anaerobic pathway comes in handy. But it's very much a sprinter, not a triathlete. If you do as many squats as you can with a heavy weight or run as fast as you can until you can go no farther, your lungs won't just tell you to stop; your muscles will start to scream bloody murder—because of the buildup of lactic acid.

Warburg, knowing all this, noticed something weird about cancer cells: they fermented glucose for energy, *even though oxygen was present.* (This feature of cancer cells is called, confusingly, aerobic glycolysis, or simply the Warburg Effect.[10]) From this discovery he inferred that cancer must develop inside the cell's power plants, later found to be mitochondria. Cancer, then, would be a disease of mitochondrial dysfunction.[11]

This was the heart of his "metabolic theory of disease," which he defended until the very end of his life. But his theory was overshadowed by a series of discoveries, including the structure of DNA in the 1950s, that led his theory's chief rival, somatic mutation theory (SMT), to prevail. Most researchers favor SMT to this day. That debate is still not settled, though. In the decades after Warburg's death in 1970, other scientists, including Pete Pedersen at Johns Hopkins, found that mitochondria inside cancer cells were indeed deformed. Recent discoveries have led some scientists to take up again the theory that Warburg first proposed.

You don't need to come down in favor of one or the other theory of cancer here. You don't even need to follow all the details in the above paragraphs. Here's the take-home lesson: Cancer cells, unlike the healthy cells in your body, *must derive most of their energy from glucose (as well as a protein called gluta-mine).* They don't have a choice. Cancer cells, in most cases at least, can't turn ketones into energy.

I bet you can guess what this means. If the healthy cells in your body can run on fat—which they can—but cancer cells need glucose or glutamine, then ketosis could be used as a smart bomb against cancer. Fasting in particular might be a double punch, since it would reduce the sugar and protein available to feed the cancer. That is, fasting may preferentially starve cancer cells and preserve healthy cells. It might not just stop some cancers in their tracks, but even prevent them in the first place.

Right now, this is a tantalizing hypothesis. Happily, there's a growing body of evidence in its favor. A leading scientific proponent of this protocol is Thomas Seyfried of Boston College. He has laid out the details in his 2013 book *Cancer as a Metabolic Disease*.[12] Earlier in his career, he was involved in testing a drug on mice that seemed to slow the growth of tumors. In studying it closely, however, he found that the drug simply lowered the appetite of the mice. That is, calorie restriction was doing the real work. He then found, based on a hunch, that some other anti-tumor drugs worked through the same mechanism.

There's plenty of evidence that caloric restriction, including fasting, can reduce tumors. One recent study put mice on three-day fasts. This appeared to help fortify healthy cells, and even sensitize cancer cells to chemotherapy, making that harsh treatment more effective.[13] Supplementation with ketones also seems to decrease "tumor cell viability" and prolong "survival of mice with metastatic cancer."[14]

Preliminary human tests suggest the benefits are not limited to the rodents.[15] Indeed, fasting may not just enhance the effects of chemo and radiation, but reduce the dreadful side-effects so many patients suffer from these treatments. Normal chemotherapy works because cancer cells grow and replicate more quickly than normal cells. So, ideally, the poison kills the cancer before it kills the patient. Not a pleasant option, but sometimes it's the best one available. When it works, the benefits just barely outweigh the costs. If the cancer recurs, however, it may then be resistant to the poison. Clearly, any therapy that can enhance the benefits and reduce the costs of chemo, radiation, and other harsh treatments would improve the ordeal for millions of cancer victims. This is why a group of scientists, including Valter Longo, whom we met in chapter 17, proposed in a 2018 article in *Nature Reviews Cancer* that doctors should add fasting-mimicking diets to their standard arsenal in their fight against cancer.[16]

How Does Fasting Protect and Heal the Body?

Fasting is part of the received wisdom of Western civilization. The Greek mathematician and philosopher Pythagoras (580–500 BC) would undergo forty-day fasts for mental clarity. Plato (427–347 BC) advised it as good medicine. And the father of medicine, Hippocrates (460–370 BC), saw it as one of the most powerful ways to restore health.

Is this just folklore? No. It's more likely the fruit of wisdom tested over centuries of practice and filtered by natural selection. For one thing, fasting—and ketosis in particular—can reduce the type of inflammation that is correlated with many autoimmune diseases, type 2 diabetes, and atherosclerosis. Research suggests that the ketone BHB (beta-hydroxybutyrate) is at least one of the key players in this process.[17]

Second, we've known for decades that modest calorie restriction can increase longevity in animals across the animal kingdom, including humans.[18] We're just now starting to study the healing powers of fasting scientifically. Still, we may already have the broad outline of how it works.

The basic theory is that fasting improves the working of networks of mitochondria (power plants) within cells, making them much more robust and efficient. Fasting can also switch parts of the cell, or the cell itself, into either repair mode or self-destruct-and-recycle mode.

Important research by a group of Harvard scientists published in *Cell Metabolism* in 2017 studied tiny nematode worms (*C. elegans*). They restricted food and genetically manipulated the worms to increase a protein called AMPK (AMP-activated kinase). A spike in AMPK tells the cell that energy supplies are low—which they would be in case of a fast. The researchers found that restricting food or genetically manipulating the worms to mimic a fast increased their life span.

Biologists like to work with nematodes because the little critters only live for two weeks, which makes them easy to study across their life span. Mice, in contrast, might hang around for a couple of years—short by human standards but glacially slow for research on a short time line.

In any case, what's this got to do with us? Well, the energy system in our cells is much like that of mice and nematodes. Our cells are highly dynamic and interconnected systems, and the mitochondria are especially so. Most cells contain thousands of mitochondria (plural for mitochondrion). And because these tiny organelles are always splitting and fusing, their shape and number can change within a cell from one moment to another.

Fasting seems to help cells maintain a healthy balance of these organelles, which could help us fight off disease. As William Mair, one of the senior authors of the Harvard study, explained:

> *Although previous work has shown how intermittent fasting can slow aging, we are only beginning to understand the underlying biology. Our work shows how crucial the plasticity of mitochondria networks is for the benefits of fasting. If we lock mitochondria in one state, we completely block the effects of fasting or dietary restriction on longevity.*[19]

In other words, our mitochondria, just like our bodies, do best when they experience bouts of feeding and fasting—rather than when they camp out at the all-you-can-eat buffet.

This is true not just for our mitochondria but also for our cells as a whole. Under the pressures of fasting, our cells start to repair themselves. In mitochondria, this is called mitophagy, and in the cell, autophagy (literally: self-eating).[20] Rather than holding on to worn-out organelles, proteins, and membranes, cells in eukaryotes (everything from yeast to humans) can recycle their parts and use them to meet their energy needs.

A lack of nutrients from food is a key trigger for this process. There are several ways this is signaled in the body. A spike in AMPK, mentioned above, is one. A drop in another protein kinase called mTOR is a second. (mTOR is a sensitive nutrient sensor.[21] The presence of just a few grams of the amino acid leucine can shut off autophagy.) A third trigger is low levels of insulin and high levels of its hormonal alter ego, glucagon. What do these signals have in common? *They're all stimulated by fasting.*

Autophagy is like a deep spring cleaning. You scrub the walls, replace your broken dishwasher, fix the leaky roof, and flush out the rain gutters. But what if a cell is beyond repair? There's an app for that too! It's called apoptosis—programmed cell death. (That sounds scary, but don't worry: you lose tens of billions of cells through apoptosis every day.) Apoptosis is like tearing down the whole house, recycling its parts, and building a new house in its place.

Cells aren't meant to live forever. They wear out, like shoes, tires, and engine blocks. Unlike shoes, tires, and engine blocks, though, cells in multi-cellular organisms are designed to schedule their own death under certain kinds of stress. Happily, they don't just rot and pollute surrounding cells. They follow a tightly regulated process that allows the body to reuse some ingredients and safely discard the waste.

Cancer cells, in contrast, ignore the Grim Reaper when he comes calling. They want to live forever. This is just one of several weird features that make cancer deadly. Cancer cells also stay stuck in the growth state and resist signals to stop. They manage to evade the immune system that could otherwise kill them. They can get the body to build blood vessels to supply them with fuel. Their genomes are unstable. And, worst of all, they spread.[22] That last feature is what usually kills cancer victims. Together, these evil superpowers make cancer one tough bugger.

But it also has an Achilles' heel: unlike healthy cells, cancer cells are stuck using the less-efficient pathway to generate energy.[23] So, to switch metaphors, cancer is like one of those evil characters from the planet Krypton who hates Superman. To fight it, we want to use anti-cancer kryptonite. That is, we want to attack cancer at its point of greatest weakness. And some of that kryptonite may come from fasting. The right kind of fasting for the right length of time may help ward off disease, starve and kill off cancerous and other severely damaged cells, and cause normal cells to repair themselves. That's a happy prospect.

Good Stress

Good stress is one of many examples of *hormesis*, which is a positive response of a cell or system to stressors. There's a truism in toxicology: The dose makes the poison. Many substances that will kill you in large amounts, like water, are harmless in small amounts. What's more, some low-level stressors actually *improve* the thing under stress.

This is one of the most ingenious traits of living organisms. Think about vaccines. They expose you to a form or dose of a toxin that is strong enough to trigger an immune response, but without causing you to contract the disease. You thus become immune to the disease itself.

The effect of radiation on the body is another (controversial) example of hormesis. Getting a direct blast of powerful gamma rays is deadly. But people exposed to low levels of ionizing radiation tend to have better health than those who don't enjoy such exposure.

For an example closer to home, consider exercise. If you lift heavy weights, you will tear muscle fibers, stress your bones, and trigger inflammation. But with the right amount of food and rest, the muscles and bones not only recover but also become stronger than they were before.

Good stress may be one of the reasons that vegetables are good for us. Virtually all plants produce natural pesticides or phytochemicals to ward off predators. These may kill bugs, but provide positive stress to our bodies, invigorating our cells, our bodies, even our minds.

Fasting is another form of good stress. Michael Mosley hints at its effect on the brain near the end of his BBC documentary on fasting. In summarizing some Alzheimer's research on mice, he observes, "It seems that fasting stresses your gray matter the way that exercise stresses your muscles." Some kinds of fasting not only induce autophagy but may induce healthy apoptosis as well.[24]

Nietzsche famously said, "That which does not kill me makes me stronger." That's not true in general. If I cut off your legs and arms but stanch the bleeding so you don't die, will you be stronger? No. Still, some forms of stress can make us stronger. Don't think of stress in itself as a bad thing. It can be good or bad, depending on the stressor, the dose, its frequency, how you respond to it, and how you think about it.

Seriously. In her great book *The Upside of Stress*, Stanford psychologist Kelly McGonigal reveals the surprising research that shows that your state of mind has a lot to do with how stress affects you.[25] If you believe a stressful event is bad for you, it probably will be. If, in contrast, you see it as a test to help you improve, it may do just that.

Of course, the right dose and sequence matter. Chronic stress without a break is a problem—and leads many of us to think we should avoid all forms of stress. If you're anxious and distracted, you may pine for a stress-free environment. When I wake up in the middle of the night, I can often put myself to sleep by imagining that I'm floating in a safe and silent tank filled with warm water. Ah. Very relaxing. But that would be a bad permanent state! We shouldn't want a zero-stress environment. If we had it, we'd end up like those tubby, bone-weakened humans in WALL-E, who have their every need met by robots and floating chaise lounges. We're designed, not as statues, but as creatures that need to experience periodic bouts of stress, followed by downtime for repair and new growth.

The Lord has created us not just to stay awake, but to switch between wakefulness and sleep. Not just to grow, but to grow and repair. Not just to exercise, but to exercise and recover. Not just to work, but to work and rest. Not just to fast, but to fast and feed.

And, every once in a while, to feast.

WEEK SIX

WEEK SIX

22

A Multi-Day Fast

You are now poised to experience the benefits of a fast for a full day and more. You may think you've *already* fasted for a full day, or at least for twenty-three hours. Isn't that almost a full day? Well, sort of. But on a 23/1 intermittent fast, like the one we did two weeks ago, you still eat every single day. And even last week—when we dropped caloric intake for the week—you ate a small meal on fast days.

To fast for a whole day—that is, to forgo all the food you normally eat during a day—you have to avoid food for about thirty-six hours, from the night before until the morning after the fast day. The good news is you're asleep for sixteen hours of it. A few weeks ago, going thirty-six hours without food may have sounded worse to you than walking on broken glass. But don't worry. If you've stuck with the program, it should be a cinch. In fact, if you're in good health, you should be able to do a forty-eight- or seventy-two-hour fast without much trouble.

The purpose of the fasting-mimicking diet is to get the benefits of a longer fast without as much work or suffering. That's why Michael Mosley took up the 5/2 fasting-mimicking diet: He found longer fasts unsustainable.

But Mosley doesn't bother to eat low-carb, let alone keto-genically, on non-fast days. If he did so, his experience might be similar to mine. When I'm in ketosis, I find it *harder* to eat one tiny meal during a fast day than just to fast for the whole day. The little meal in the evening seems to kick-start my ap-petite. It's even worse if I try to eat something in the morning as Mosley does. That seems to confuse my body into expecting a feast day. This is common for those who fast while in ketosis. At some point, you may find the same thing. In fact, you can test out the question this week, since you'll be fasting for at least thirty-six hours.

As in previous weeks, you should restrict the hours when you eat to no more than eight hours during the day (except for Sunday). And on Monday, Tuesday, and Wednesday, you should hew strictly to keto-friendly foods with plenty of natural fat. You want to be deep into ketosis by Thursday, when you'll do a thirty-six- to seventy-two-hour fast. That is, one to three full days.

You might think that a seventy-two-hour fast would be twice as hard as a thirty-six-hour fast. But for many people, fast-ing gets easier after forty-eight hours. Even during the first forty-eight hours, though, your hunger will wax and wane. It will not get more and more intense.

You should pack your schedule with all the spiritual prac-tices you can manage. It will not only enrich the fast. It will help fill the extra time when you would be preparing and eating food.

How long should you go? As long as the only thing you

experience is hunger, and you don't start feeling nauseated or sick, but no longer than seventy-two hours. If you're worried about your blood sugar, you should check it periodically. (And if you're diabetic, you should be under a doctor's care when trying this.)

Whenever you break your fast, be sure to do it slowly. Your insulin and blood sugar will be low. Your ketones will be high. Your stomach may have shrunk, and your body will be producing less digestive acid. In fact, much of your G/I tract may be taking a nap. Start with some soup or bone broth, then some vegetables, then meat and all the rest. In fact, you can simply follow the order of a multi-course meal: soup, salad, entrée with vegetables, dessert. Just spread out the first two dishes to give your system time to warm up.

The really nice way to break a long fast is with a special feast. For more on how to celebrate a feast, see chapter 28.

23

Fasting Together

Fasts, like feasts, have historically been communal acts, tied to special days and seasons. So why have I mostly treated fasting as an individual discipline? Well, this is a book, and individuals read books. Also, in an age when Catholics and Protestants are rarely obliged to fast, any revival of fasting will have to start somewhere. No group project can succeed unless the members of the group put forth effort. And if individuals don't freely invest in a corporate fast, it becomes a mere external ritual.

Fasting may begin with the solitary self, but it should not end there. If fasting is good for our bodies, then it should also be good for the Body of Christ on Earth. In fact, I suspect that we can only fully experience its spiritual power when we do it together—as families, congregations, and as the whole Church.

So how do we take a private spiritual practice and make it a joint effort? How do we turn it into a popular movement? Although these questions merit a whole book, here are a few suggestions.

Getting Started

First, a warning: Don't badger your spouse, children, friends, fellow churchgoers, and co-workers into fasting. This is a bad way to plant seeds of interest. Instead, adopt a fasting lifestyle yourself and then pray for opportunities to tell others about it. If you've spent several months making fasting a permanent part of your life, people will notice.

But they need to notice in the right way. Remember, Jesus warned his followers not to put on a show when fasting. Instead, he told them to try to appear not to be fasting (Matt. 6:16–18). If you look pale and bedraggled, you *might* get the sympathy points you'd hoped for, but that will be your only reward. Or, if you make a show of it, you might get no sympathy but instead repel others who might otherwise think about fasting. As St. Josemaría Escrivá put it, "Choose mortifications that don't mortify others."[1] To fast properly you have to pass through the horns of a dilemma: You need to inspire interest in fasting without talking and complaining about it. Trust me. If you do it right, curious friends and family will ask about it in due time.

Preset corporate fasts are one way around this dilemma. For one thing, group fasts reduce the dangers Jesus warned about. If everyone around you is fasting, you're much less likely to feel self-righteous or try to make a show of it.

Also, if enough people are involved, families and businesses orient themselves around the fast. Those in your social circle aren't treating you like a weirdo and tempting you to break the fast. Instead, they help to reinforce the fast with positive peer pressure.

Fasting as a Family

We already know that feasts are family affairs. We go out of our way to be with our family at Christmas and Easter. That's why the days around Thanksgiving are the busiest travel days of the year. Since feasting is the yin to the yang of fasting, it's hardly a stretch to make fasting a family affair as well. And since family is the first society, family fasting is a natural place to start when it comes to corporate fasting.

Of course, you'll need agreement from your family members for this to work. (Remember the warning above.) And the details will differ from family to family. Small children are usually exempt from fasting because they're growing and need plenty of calories. That doesn't mean they should be excluded. If your family includes young children, you can tailor the details to the individual. The basic rule (assuming no one is elderly or in poor health) is, *the older the family member, the more stringent the fast.*

Take, for instance, the Ember Days fasts (which we'll discuss later). Perhaps you and your spouse choose to do a water-only fast on those days; older teenagers limit their eating to one to four hours; and younger children give up sweets and other things they like to eat but can live without. Remember, a fast is supposed to be a sacrifice, not torture.

The same system will work for every other corporate fast—Wednesdays and Fridays, Advent, Lent, and so forth. Just be sure to talk as a family about the proper reasons for fasting, and to incorporate special family prayers during the fast.

For instance, following Ezra's example, you should pray together for protection. When Ezra led a group of Jewish exiles back to Israel from Babylon, he called on them to fast and pray to God for "a safe journey for ourselves, our children, and all our possessions." They did so, Ezra writes, and God "listened to our entreaty" (Ezra 8:21–23).

Solid research confirms the cliché that "the family that prays together stays together."[2] If done right, fasting can supercharge both the binding and the protective power of family prayer.

Fasting as a Congregation

For years, Jentezen Franklin, Senior Pastor of the multi-site Free Chapel Worship Center in Gainesville, Georgia, has been leading his congregation on a twenty-one-day fast at the beginning of each year. Franklin took inspiration from the Old Testament prophet Daniel.

At the beginning of the book of Daniel, Nebuchadnezzar brings the prophet-to-be, his three companions, and some other young Israelites to Babylon. The king tells his eunuch to prepare the group to appear before the king by feeding them the same rich food and drink the king enjoys. Daniel, no doubt because of Jewish dietary laws, does not want to defile himself with this food, and asks the eunuch if he can just eat vegetables instead. The eunuch objects, "I fear lest my lord the king, who appointed your food and your drink, should see that you were in poorer condition than the youths who are of your own age. So you would endanger my head with the king."

Daniel proposes a solution for himself and his companions: a temporary vegan diet. "Test your servants for ten days," he says, "let us be given vegetables to eat and water to drink. Then let our appearance and the appearance of the youths who eat the king's rich food be observed by you, and according to what you see deal with your servants." The eunuch agrees. After the ten days, the men look better than those who have eaten the king's food. "So the steward took away their rich food and the wine they were to drink," we're told, "and gave them vegetables" (Dan. 1:1–17).

The twenty-one-day veggie diet mimics another abstinence that Daniel undertakes much later in life, under the Persian king Cyrus. This time Daniel is praying and eating only vegetables as a period of mourning for the plight of his people. After three weeks of this, an angel appears to him. Daniel learns that the angel had tried to come to his aid on the first day of the fast, but the demon in charge of Persia had withstood him. Finally, on the twenty-first day, the archangel Michael shows up to battle the demon, thereby freeing the lower-ranking angel to come to Daniel to reveal to him some things that will happen in the future (Dan. 10).

This is one of the most vivid biblical accounts of the warfare that takes place in the spiritual realm. Angels fight a powerful demon, and the prayer and fasting of a holy prophet plays a key role in helping the angels overcome the demon. Does this mean everyone who prays and goes vegan for three weeks will receive prophetic words from an archangel? No. In fact, Daniel's practice isn't really a model for a general fast—despite the popularity of the "Daniel Fast" in Christian circles. First of all, it's really abstinence rather than fasting. Eating a veggie diet for a few weeks might be a good idea,[3] and it might be part of a longer seasonal fast such as Lent. But going vegan for a stretch isn't, strictly speaking, a fast.

Still, for a non-fasting church, it could be a step in the right direction. I have no doubt that a church that adopts this practice at the beginning of every year will find that the practice bears fruit. Why? Not because there's a simple formula to get God to bless us. We can't dictate the terms. Rather, it's because spiritual sacrifices, pursued for the right reasons, have some positive effect. "God is committed to rewarding those acts of the human heart that signify human helplessness and hope in God," notes John Piper.[4]

In his book *Fasting*, Jentezen Franklin writes about the many blessings and miracles that have resulted over the years in his community from this effort.[5] Church members are invited to participate as much as they can. Some do water-only fasts for three weeks. Some do that for a few days and then switch to a vegetable diet. Others follow a vegetable diet the whole time as Daniel did. The key thing is that it is a congregation-wide effort.

Church fasting campaigns tend to take place in independent—especially charismatic—evangelical churches. Their pastors tend to have a lot of autonomy—for good or ill—to lead fasting campaigns. If you don't attend one of these churches, you may never have experienced a congregational fast. But there's no reason such fasts should be limited to independent churches—somebody just has to get things started.

In Jentezen Franklin's church, it started with him. Surely, pastors of most churches—Catholic or Protestant—can *encourage* their congregations to join in corporate, that is church-wide, fasts.

Of course, Franklin had already fasted for years before he launched a church-wide campaign. What are interested laypeople to do if their pastor doesn't really fast, let alone encourage fasting? Well, the effort can start at the grassroots with the parishioners themselves. Beyond family, the most natural unit for a group fast is the local congregation or parish. Many Christians are already involved in small groups, which may gather for prayer, reading, and socializing. If you can gain interest among friends and family, start a prayer *and fasting* circle. Or incorporate fasting into a pre-existing prayer group. You could start by studying the case for fasting. You might even—ahem—read this book together. You could also meet with your pastoral staff and talk to them about what you're doing. Heck, a fasting-averse pastor might reconsider the question if many of his flock are fasting on their own.

Fasting with the Universal Church

Ideally, a local church will act in concert with the whole Body of Christ. Perhaps the best way to do this is to follow the feasts and fasts of the traditional Christian calendar. Most local churches already recognize Advent/Christmas and Lent/Easter, so it's not that hard to focus as a congregation on those long fasting seasons.[6] And though they are less common, the Ember Days are also fixed on the calendar.

These fasts are the subject of the next chapter.

24

Fasting and the Christian Year

It was hard to be a Catholic in 2018. Starting in the summer, every week brought a new story about sex abuse and cover-ups by the Church hierarchy. First came the Pennsylvania attorney general's report, which revealed decades of abuse and cover-up, involving some three hundred priests. Yes, most of the violations had taken place decades earlier, but that was cold comfort.

Then came the appalling revelations of Cardinal Theodore McCarrick. McCarrick was for many years archbishop of the powerful archdiocese of Washington, DC—where I live. Even in retirement, he still played a key role in the course of Church events. Especially worrisome, Archbishop Carlo Maria Viganò, a former apostolic nuncio to the US, published the first of three explosive letters claiming that Pope Francis knew about McCarrick's predations and the informal restrictions placed on him by Pope Benedict XVI but made McCarrick a highly trusted advisor nonetheless. Later developments made it clear that, despite the angry tone of Viganò's first letter, his core claim was true.

It was enough to cast many devout Catholics into despair.

The dithering and ineffectual responses of many otherwise-faithful bishops made it even more painful. I was reminded of the lines from the poem "The Second Coming" by W. B. Yeats: "The best lack all conviction, while the worst / Are full of passionate intensity."

But God can and does turn even great evils into greater goods. "The darker the night, the brighter the stars, the deeper the grief, the closer is God!" Dostoyevsky wrote in *Crime and Punishment*. The spiritual darkness and grief inspired many calls for spiritual renewal and a recovery of ancient spiritual disciplines. For instance, on August 18, 2018, Madison, Wisconsin, Bishop Robert Morlino wrote a powerful letter decrying "all the sins of sexual depravity committed by members of the clergy and episcopacy."[1] He offered a public Mass of Reparation on September 14. He also kept the traditional Ember Days fasts near the end of September and invited the Catholic faithful in his diocese to do the same.

If you heard about this, did you think: *Ember what?* I might have thought the same, except that I happened to be working on this book and had stumbled upon this tradition in my research.

What Are Ember Days?

Ember Days were communal fasts that Christians held four times a year at the beginning of the four seasons. "Ember" doesn't refer to burning coals—though that image seems apt these days. It's from the Anglo-Saxon *ymbren*, meaning a circle or revolution, which may itself be a corruption of the Latin phrase *quatuor tempora*, meaning "four times."

We don't know just when these fasts started in Christian history. The prophet Zechariah does mention four fasts and feasts in Israel, which may be a precursor (Zech. 8:1). We do know this: Already by the fourth century Christians in Rome were keeping Ember Days. It was only in the eleventh century, though, that Pope Gregory VII fixed the dates in the liturgical calendar.

These fasts were so common by the thirteenth century that when St. Thomas Aquinas wrote about fasting in his *Summa Theologiae*, he mentioned two fasts: Lent and Ember Days.

Think of these as seasonal reboots of your spiritual life. They are fixed times set aside to pray, thank God for his abundant blessings, identify with Christ's suffering, help the needy, and renew the spirit of repentance from sin. Shouldn't we do these things every day? Of course. Because we are all fallen, however, we tend to grow lax in doing the things we ought to do every day. That's why it helps to have special, scheduled times to awaken us from our sloth and boredom.

Where Did They Go?

So, what happened to Ember Days? As you might have guessed, they were a casualty of the 1960s. The bishops of the Second Vatican Council retained them but thought local dioceses should have more flexibility to set the dates. After all, seasons vary in the northern and southern hemispheres. In Argentina, for instance, Christmas comes at the beginning of their summer. Surely fasts fixed to earthly seasons should take account of this local diversity.

In light of this, St. Pope Paul VI handed the scheduling of

Ember Days over to national bishops' conferences, who, for the most part, dropped the ball. The US bishops never got around to picking dates, which meant that the fasts went the way of rotary dial phones.

Some older die-hards still keep these fasts in their private lives. Most of those who came of age after the 1960s have never even heard of them.

Recovery

Until 2018. The crisis in the Church had many Catholics searching for solutions. There was an overwhelming sense that in a desire to be hip and modern, too many—especially many in the Church hierarchy—had abandoned truths and practices that, if anything, we should have been doubling down on.

Bishop Morlino had the right impulse. Rather than counsel despair, he called the faithful back to a long-standing practice that was abandoned about the time things really started to go off the rails. I doubt that's a coincidence.

Morlino wasn't the only one. At the same moment, Catholic blogs and websites started mentioning the Ember Days.

Great minds think alike and all that.

Try It. It's Not that Hard.

So, what's involved? The Ember Days are three days of fasting, only two of which are consecutive. As we've mentioned, Catholics universally abstained from meat on Friday until, well, the 1960s. And for many centuries, they fasted on Wednesday and Friday. The Ember Days just add one day, Saturday, to what used to be a weekly custom. In fall 2018, the dates were Wednesday, September 19; Friday, September 21; and Saturday, September 22. These were the first Ember Days fasts I ever kept. I happened to be speaking at a conference in South Carolina. I also had had a serious stomach bug the previous Monday, when I ate nothing. So my inaugural Ember Days were more challenging that they might have been.

As usual, the fasts are really abstinences. You're not expected to give up food all day—or even to eat fewer meals. To follow the pre-1960s custom, you just need to eat less than you normally would for two meals, while giving up meat (the flesh of land animals) that would otherwise leave you feeling satisfied. You still get to eat one normal-size meal with meat. Only on Friday would you abstain from all land animal meat and eat only fish.

Honestly, given our current crisis in the Church, this seems lame. This tradition seems like a perfect chance to integrate a fasting-mimicking diet into our fasting routine, four times a year. Try eating only one small meal a day on the Ember Days. Remember that it should be only one-fourth of your regular calorie consumption (about five hundred calories for women; six hundred for men).

As with the fasting-mimicking diet, you still won't have to go all day without eating, but you'll spend most of the time during those days in a fasted state. And your total consumption will be so low that you will gain many of the benefits of an even longer fast.

My meal of choice? Guacamole made with two avocados, with lime, salt, and salsa, with some cucumber slices, eaten a few hours before bedtime.

Lent and Advent

The secular world celebrates Christmas, one of the two high points of the Christian year. Why is this? In part because even the most secular Western society still has vestiges of a Christian past. It may also be because this holiday ("holy day") is a good excuse to buy and sell food and gifts. But it's also because Christmas is a feast, and who doesn't like a feast?

The high point of the Christian Year—Easter—gets short shrift compared to Christmas.[2] But traditions such as candy and the Easter bunny persist—making it the other moment in the Christian year that still shapes the calendar throughout the Western world.

The world passes over in silence the two periods that precede Christmas and Easter—Advent and Lent. In fact, department stores and pop culture start plugging Christmas at the beginning of Advent, just after Thanksgiving, even though Christmas doesn't start until December 25, and continues until Epiphany—after most folks have set their Christmas tree out on the curb.

When Christmas greetings turn up in the middle of Advent, Catholics and other Christians who follow the liturgical calendar complain that everyone's doing it wrong. They're technically right: Christmas hasn't yet come! Still, this is a losing battle, at least for the wider secular world. That's because Lent and Advent are both traditional seasons of fasting. There's no clear financial incentive for Amazon, Walmart, and Starbucks to push fasting, abstinence, and penance for two and a half months every year.

Besides, most people just don't like to fast. We'd much prefer to get straight to the feast. Unless we get a Third Great Awakening that turns believers back to the deep practices of Christian history, I wouldn't hold my breath waiting for Safeway to spend marketing dollars urging customers to eat far less than they normally do for two out of the twelve months of the year.

At Advent and Lent we reenact, every year, the moment when Christ was born on Earth as a baby, and when he died for our sins and rose from the dead. Advent is more about waiting with excitement. We sing songs like "O Come, O Come, Emmanuel" and "Come, Thou Long Expected Jesus." Lent is more about repentance and entering into the suffering of Jesus. Still, both are times to prepare for God's coming.

Surely these moments are worth preparing for. And since Christmas and Easter are the two greatest feasts of the Christian Year, it's fitting that the greatest fasts of the year should precede them.

Alas, at the moment, only the Eastern traditions still retain robust fasts during these periods. Should Protestants and Catholics adopt one of the Eastern fasts—which vary from one region to another? That would be better than what we're doing now. Still, I doubt there's one best way to keep the Advent and Lenten fasts. Any detailed, universal fast would risk appearing arbitrary. Remember how the meaning of eating land animals changed over time and place? Since the Eastern fasts have persisted for so long, though, we could do much worse than to follow them. For much of Orthodox Lent, for instance, the faithful eat a vegan diet. This may give your gut a rest, switch your body into repair and recovery mode, and have other physical and spiritual perks that we have not yet discovered.

Based on what we've learned about the health benefits of intermittent fasting, we could also limit the amount of time when we eat to a shorter than normal period. Maybe, after you've locked in the fasting lifestyle, you frequently limit your eating to an eight-hour time window on most days. During Advent and Lent, then, you might shrink that window to six, four, or even one hour on most days.

A few weeks ago, you probably would have balked at that suggestion. But if you've stuck with the plan in this book, you've already prepared yourself for a fasting season that lasts about six weeks in the case of Lent and five weeks in the case of Advent. You've also acquired the skill of limiting the amount of time when you eat. You now have what it takes to make the two greatest fasting seasons of the Christian year part of your fasting lifestyle.

We know that God wants us to fast and pray. So, does that mean that the Church should mandate Advent and Lenten fasting, specifying what and when to eat? I doubt that would improve things—and it seems unlikely to happen in any case. But there's an alternative: What if millions of faithful laity and clergy decided to start fasting, at least partially, one or two days of every week? What if we chose to keep a fast for three days, four times a year? What if, all over our world, Christians *freely* started marking Advent and Lent with fasting? What if the Church encouraged this, without requiring details? What if Christians of all stripes suddenly took up these practices and prayed in unison, as Christ prayed in John 17? What would happen if we channeled our extra time and hunger into fervent prayers to the Lord to renew his Church and to deliver us from evil?

We'll never know unless we try.[3]

25

What About Longer Fasts?

In the 1990s Dr. Bill Bright, founder of Campus Crusade for Christ, felt God call him to do a forty-day fast. "Increasingly I have been gripped with a growing sense of urgency to call upon God to send revival to our beloved country," he wrote. "In the spring and summer of 1994, I had a growing conviction that God wanted me to fast and pray for forty days for revival in America and for the fulfillment of the Great Commission in obedience to our Lord's command."[1]

Three weeks into his fast, he felt called to pray for two million Christians in North America to undertake the same forty-day fast. He soon wrote a book and launched a fasting crusade nationwide.[2] Before long, other prominent evangelicals such as Pat Robertson had signed on. In 1997, eight hundred evangelical leaders met in Dallas to further the cause. By 1998, even the *New York Times* was reporting on the movement.

"Fasting and prayer is the atomic bomb, or the hydrogen bomb, of all the Christian disciplines," Bright said in the *Times* story. "Prayer has great power, but fasting with prayer has infinitely more power."[3]

I don't know if two million American Christians fasted for forty days before the turn of the millennium. I do know that Bright helped make fasting popular in evangelical circles for several years—even among some who had never fasted before.

In 1997 my wife and I, along with some friends, decided to fast all day every Sunday. (We didn't know that Sunday is supposed to be a feast day. Oh well.) We managed to do it for a few months, until summer came.

This was the only time I had fasted for twenty-four hours. It was a tough slog. We were hungry all day. It felt like all cost and no benefit—except for the weight loss, which I didn't need. As a result, it never became a habit. I now realize that this was in large part because we were eating an extremely low-fat, high-carb diet during the rest of the week. It made a one-day fast dreary, and a forty-day fast unthinkable.

Reinforcing this opinion was an experience I had had a few years before: I witnessed someone endure a forty-day fast.

After college, I had spent two wonderful years at Asbury Seminary. (This is where I met my wife, Ginny.) A fellow student who lived next door, named Bill (no relation to Bill Bright), decided to embark on a forty-day fast. Mind you, this was not a water-only fast. Bill drank generous amounts of fruit juice throughout the day. As the days and weeks dragged on, I watched him grow ever paler and weaker. He couldn't concentrate. He couldn't exercise. Climbing the three flights of stairs to our floor was a burden. He didn't seem to walk so much as to drag his legs along for the journey. And although he lost over twenty-five pounds, he looked less lean when he ended the fast than when he started it—no doubt because he was losing lean muscle mass. I don't remember if he made it to forty days. What I do remember is my conclusion: A forty-day fast is crazy. I would not have tried it unless Jesus appeared to me in person and told me to do so.

I'm not sure where my fellow student Bill got the idea to drink juice. But Bill Bright suggested a similar routine, following the plan of Bolivian evangelist Dr. Julio C. Ruibal. Here's the schedule he recommended:

5:00 a.m.–8:00 a.m.
- Fruit juices, preferably freshly squeezed or blended and diluted in 50 percent distilled water if the fruit is acidic. Apple, pear, grapefruit, papaya, watermelon, or other fruit juices are generally preferred. If you cannot do your own juicing, buy juices without sugar or additives.

10:30 a.m.–noon
- Fresh vegetable juice made from lettuce, celery, and carrots in three equal parts.

2:30 p.m.–4:00 p.m.
- Herbal tea with a drop of honey. Avoid black tea or any tea with caffeine.

6:00 p.m.–8:30 p.m.
- Broth made from boiling potatoes, celery, and carrots with no salt. After boiling about half an hour, pour the water into a container and drink it.[4]

The problems with this method are legion. Feeding is spread out over fifteen and half hours, and the diet gets its calories from liquid sugar and boiled potatoes. Bright may not have realized that this would be a problem, since many people think that if juice doesn't have "added sugar," then it's low sugar. In truth, juice is mainly sugar removed from its natural matrix of soluble fiber. There's no good reason to extract the sugar from fruit and vegetables before ingesting them. If you want fruit and vegetables, eat them.

Also, he may not have known that boiled potatoes quickly turn to sugar.

To add insult to injury, he advised fasters to avoid black tea, caffeine, and salt, which he thought could stimulate the appetite.

Finally, he discouraged exercise, except for a short daily prayer walk.

This is a really bad way to endure a forty-day fast. For most people, it would involve a daily calorie deficit but without a single full-day fast. It gets over 90 percent of its calories from sugar— most of it in liquid form; it contains almost no fat or protein; and it keeps the feeding window open for most of one's waking hours. For an insulin-resistant person, this would encourage the body to slow down, store fat, and use lean body mass. Avoiding exercise, especially resistance training, would make this problem worse.

It would even be possible to *gain body fat* on this fast, since no serving sizes are recommended. If a 125-pound woman drank 2,500 calories from juice every day for forty days straight, but got precious little protein or fat, she would likely end up weaker, heavier, and more insulin resistant than when she started. Maybe she would reap spiritual benefits from the discipline. But as a fasting method that takes body, mind, and soul into account, a liquid sugar "fast" is a dreadful prospect.

This is a recurring danger with fasting fads: They start with a burst of enthusiasm led by a popular figure. They draw energy from emotion, skip centuries of Christian wisdom on fasting, and fail to incorporate well-founded scientific evidence on the effects of fasting. They may even incorporate nutrition myths such as the idea of juice cleanses. At some point, they peter out as the excitement fades and reality sets in.

I believe God inspired Bill Bright to fast and to call other Christians to do the same. I'm thankful that he helped evangelicals overcome resistance to fasting. But God clearly didn't provide the details. Bright said himself that he adopted the diet from Julio Ruibal. Ruibal was a leading charismatic figure in Latin America who was tragically murdered by a drug cartel in Colombia in 1996. Bright identified him as a "nutritionist," but Ruibal had no training in nutrition, so far as I can tell. And he could not have known about the physical effects of fasting that we've discovered over the last twenty years. My guess is that Bright picked up on the juicing fad that was popular in the 1990s and thought it would help with fasting.

Like Bill Bright, I, too, felt called to write a book on fasting, though I haven't received any precise messages from the Holy Spirit (alas—it would have made it a lot easier to write this book!). That's no surprise. God rarely gives us detailed marching orders beyond what we can find in Scripture, perennial Church teaching, and good spiritual counsel bathed in prayer and fasting. When we go beyond that, we're tempted to identify what we feel passionately about with the will of God, and even make things up on the fly as if they have a divine stamp of approval. That's a dangerous temptation.

We already know that God wants us to fast. Beyond that, he has given us minds and evidence, and he expects us to use them. Fasting is hard, and it can be risky if not done right. It involves the body, mind, and soul—the whole person in his totality. For fasting to become a widespread, sustainable, and helpful practice for Christians, it needs to be rooted, not in fads, fleeting emotions, and private revelations, but in Scripture, time-tested practice, the Christian calendar, and sound science.

How Long?

We still haven't addressed the question: Should you fast for more than three days straight? What about a week? How about two weeks, or even forty days? Do longer fasts promise greater spiritual and physical bounty? Or do the costs outweigh the benefits?

There's no simple answer, beyond the truism that longer fasts are harder, and riskier, than shorter ones. Both research and clinical experience confirm the claim that, for many fasters, hunger subsides after seventy-two hours. So, if you can make it three days, have enough body fat, and can keep your electrolytes balanced, you can probably make it much longer.

There's a case to be made for a five-day fast every once in a while: As we noted earlier, our resting energy expenditure goes up for three days during a complete fast, and only returns to its baseline after day five. So if you're healthy, you could do a water-only fast for that length of time without slowing down your metabolism. Another study shows that growth hormone was still higher than baseline in subjects at the end of a five-day fast.[5]

That might suggest that five days is a sweet spot, except that this might just be an artifact of the studies. That is, most of the careful research on fasting has been limited to five days—like the study mentioned above. Recall that Valter Longo's fasting-mimicking diet lasts for five days.

For evidence from longer fasts, we have to turn to studies of Ramadan—Muslims' monthlong daily intermittent fast—and to clinical reports. TrueNorth Health Center in California, for instance, has been putting people on two-week, water-only fasts for the past thirty years. In some cases, they go as long as forty days. They have the testimony of about ten thousand people who have been through one of their programs, some of whom I've met. They have used these monitored regimens to treat obesity, high blood pressure, diabetes, autoimmune disorders, and more.[6]

Jason Fung and others have helped patients reverse obesity and type 2 diabetes with fasts as long as seven to fourteen days.

Longevity researchers such as Valter Longo and Luigi Fontana think that multi-week fasts may hold promise for cell repair and fighting cancer. Fontana predicts that someday, doctors may advise two- to three-week fasts once every five years for health. At the moment, though, all we have are anecdotes. "There are still a lot of unanswered questions," Fontana admits. "But based on what we know, taking in calories all day is not healthy."[7]

Heck, maybe a forty-day calorie-free fast holds secrets for body and soul. Still, at the moment, it seems extreme and unnecessary. Based on what we know, eight five-day fasts spread over a year may very well provide most of the upside to a forty-day fast, without the downside risks.

In the meantime, we should get serious about the (roughly) forty-day Christian seasons of partial fasts—especially since fasts are much more likely to be communal during these times. They're punctuated by mini-feasts on Sunday, which should help to keep our metabolisms from grinding to a halt. And both Advent and Lent end with great feasts.

Perhaps we should take a cue from Eastern Churches, who

during Advent and Lent limit their meat consumption during the week and focus on vegetables. This is, in effect, a fast not only from sugar and simple carbs, but from protein as well. Recall the fasting-mimicking diet that we discussed in chapter 17? Its benefits come from reducing protein consumption, which signals cells to go into repair and recycle mode.

As mentioned earlier, during Advent and Lent you might also choose to limit the time window for eating more strictly than you normally do.

Another possibility would be a "fat fast," which Jason Fung sometimes prescribes for patients who have a hard time getting started with fasting.[8] This is pretty much what it sounds like: a super-ketogenic diet. You restrict your eating entirely to very-high-fat foods. As you might guess, this suppresses the appetite, encourages low insulin levels and blood sugar, and boosts ketones. Just what you want when you're fasting.

Or, perhaps you could mix the fat fast with some vegetables but lay off the meat and other protein.

There are lots of options. You now have enough experience with different kinds of fasts to experiment for yourself. Just be sure to apply what you've learned in this book. Don't make longer fasts harder, and less helpful, than they should be. For instance, if you try a water-only fast for a week or longer, you should not be underweight when you start, and you should talk to your doctor first. No matter what you choose, *avoid* fruit juice fasts. Eating whole, especially green, vegetables is one thing. Chugging sugar water is quite another. The first matches our design plan. The second matches our own recent, and ill-considered, designs.

The Body's Grand Design

We are created by God in his image. We are also fallen creatures in need of spiritual healing. This dual understanding of man has served as a rubric as we explore how best to eat, fast, and feast. It's informed every page of this book. We should know, however, that it contradicts a cherished modern story, one that reaches deep into our culture.

According to this story, the stunningly intricate designs of life—from the mammalian eye, heart, and immune system, to our integrated metabolisms and the information-processing inside cells—aren't what they seem. The "design" is an illusion. All life, including human life, is pointless happenstance.

Sure, everyone concedes that organisms *look* designed. As arch-atheist Richard Dawkins famously put it in his book *The Blind Watchmaker*, "Biology is the study of complicated things that give the appearance of having been designed for a purpose."[1] Note that phrase "give the appearance of." Behind Dawkins's statement lies Charles Darwin. In 1859, the British naturalist proposed in his *On the Origin of Species* that life's amazing adaptation is really the result of a blind sifting process he called natural selection.

Here's the basic idea: Some members of a species have a survival advantage over others. As a result, they produce more offspring, and their traits get passed on and come to predominate. At one level, to grasp this idea of "survival of the fittest" is to believe it. If the organism that leaves the most offspring among its kin is "fittest," then the fittest will indeed survive.

But Darwin didn't merely suggest that natural selection explains some minor features of populations that already exist. He argued that natural selection (with some other minor processes) could account for life's manifest design, without any recourse to purpose, God, design, or whatever. In the 1930s, Darwin's theory was combined with genetics to become "Neo-Darwinism," which identifies genetic mutations as the source of change. These mutations are random in the sense that they don't happen on purpose to help the organism survive. This idea soon became entrenched in biology—so entrenched that many Christian academics do their best to work it into their theology.

If you spend any time reading the literature on human diet and nutrition, you encounter this view. Authors use it to spin all sorts of stories. We were not created in God's image to be fruitful and multiply and fill the earth and subdue it, they tell us. Rather, we're a passing stage of a blind process of differential survival, reproduction, and chance.

Darwin's conjecture has become the main prop for modern materialism. This view holds that matter and energy are the ultimate reality. Things like consciousness, purpose, and religious beliefs are just so much froth on the mindless churning of molecules.

But matter is a poor candidate for ultimate reality. We've known for almost a century that the universe had a beginning. *It has an age.* We've also known for several decades that the laws and constants of our universe are finely tuned to allow for life, to a degree of precision that boggles the mind. Together these twin discoveries strongly suggest creation. As Nobel-Prize-winning physicist Arno Penzias said, "Astronomy leads us to a unique event, a universe which was created out of nothing, one with the very delicate balance needed to provide exactly the conditions required to permit life, and one which has an underlying (one might say 'supernatural') plan."[2]

In the face of these findings, the materialist is reduced to positing countless unobserved universes just to explain away the origin and fine-tuning of this one. Or to claiming, as the late Stephen Hawking did, that "the universe can and will create itself from nothing."[3] Let that sink in. It is truly materialism's reduction to the absurd.

But what about biology? Do we have good reason to believe in the sweeping power of Darwin's mechanism? Could it really have generated all the life forms we see around us? No. The evidence points in the opposite direction: Beyond the borders of an organism's diverse population, selection-and-mutation soon hit a brick wall. If an adaptive change needs more than two coordinated mutations to succeed, it won't happen, however generous you are with the time window.[4] Any major innovation would require far, far more mutations.

It's not clear that even *directed* mutations could turn one organism into another. Thousands of years of dog breeding, for instance, have never given rise to a new species.

Darwin's theory lives on for at least four reasons.

First, it explains a few things well, such as modest adaptations within species and genera.

Second, it's so supple that it can explain both adaptation and its opposite, dysfunction. If something works well, then that's the wunderkind we call natural selection. If something appears substandard, then that's Darwinism too. It's a trial-and-error process after all! Most who invoke such explanations don't pause to notice that these just-so stories are painfully short on details. The stories also have proven wrong in some spectacular cases. "Junk DNA," for instance, turned out not to be junk at all. Darwinists assumed it was evolutionary detritus. Intelligent design proponents predicted that most "junk DNA" would prove to have important functions. It has.

Third, the history of science shows that dominant paradigms tend to hang on long after the evidence has turned against them. Scientists have their careers invested in them, after all. This tendency for a theory to hang on in the face of mounting contrary evidence can be especially true of theories focused on events in the distant past, since they are hard to test in the way one could test a theory in, say, experimental chemistry.

A final reason the theory persists is that it props up the worldview of materialism. Without it, atheism is in trouble (as Richard Dawkins himself admitted), so Darwinists cling to it fiercely and punish dissenters in the academy.[5]

What Natural Selection Can Explain

Of course, natural selection explains *some* things. Our best example of its power is antibiotic resistance in bacteria. If you have billions of harmful bacteria in your feverish body and flood it with an antibiotic, one bacterium may have a quirk in its outer membrane that gives it a resistance to the drug. The drug kills off all its cousins that lack this advantage. Then the resistant bug multiplies to fill the ecosystem that is your body. (A bacterium reproduces not sexually but by splitting into two identical daughter cells—so you just need one to get started.)

Despite huge populations and superfast reproductive times, however, they never become anything more than humble bacteria. Moreover, such mutations exact a fitness cost. The resistant strain of bacteria has an advantage against an antibiotic, but not because it has evolved a superpower. Rather, it has *lost* something that just happens to give it an advantage in that odd environment. When the antibiotic-resistant bacteria must compete with the ordinary strain of bacteria absent the antibiotic drug, the ordinary strain wins.

What's going on here? The problem is not just "that random mutation and natural selection are grossly inadequate to *build* complex structures," argues biochemist Michael Behe, "they strongly tend to *break* them." As a result, and a bit paradoxically, Darwin's process can "help form new species and new genera, but chiefly by promoting the *loss* of genetic abilities. Over time, dwindling degradatory options fence in an evolutionary lineage, halting organismal change before it crosses the family line."[6]

For instance, imagine a lush tropical island that is peaceful near the ground but buffeted by very high winds starting about thirty feet above the ground. A mutant bird may be born on the island without wings. This poor bird lacks something:

namely, flight-worthy wings. But on this island, being flightless is an advantage, since there are no predators of flightless birds. And so, over time, all the birds that can fly may be blown out to sea, leaving behind cute wingless kiwi-like birds reproducing after their kind.

This is just a thought experiment—like so much of Darwinian theory—but it captures the evidence for natural selection. You can't build new organisms with new features—let alone the whole biosphere!—just by breaking and removing parts from older ones. Darwin's mechanism can preserve the fittest members of a population. It can tweak around the edges. As others have said, it can explain the survival of the fittest but not the arrival of the fittest. It's a filter, not a creator. It can't create new systems, organs, and types of organisms. It can't account for the deep design of living things.

Scientist Doug Axe argues in his powerful book *Undeniable* that we should trust our sense that life is what it appears to be: a grand design vastly beyond our ken.[7] We build machines from the outside using separate and unrelated parts. Organisms, in contrast, develop from the inside toward a goal in a staggering feat of unity and integration. If all goes as planned, a single-celled human embryo the size of a poppy seed becomes a fully developed newborn baby in nine months.

The fact that so many clever people explain away life's stunning design is not the fault of the evidence. It's the fault of a theory that induces blindness in its adherents. Christians, who believe in a personal God, need not be cowed into denying the design of life. For those with eyes to see, the conclusion is unavoidable: whatever the details of life's history and complexity, mutation and natural selection are not the main characters.

Am I saying we can or should deduce the details of biology from theology? No. Am I advising us to reject "evolution" in every sense of that word? No. I am saying that our thinking should be integrated. When we remove the blinders and allow the evidence of nature to inform our theology, and vice versa, we emerge with a better framework to understand and explore the world and ourselves.

So What?

What does all this have to do with fasting? A lot. If you assume that everything about us is the fruit of Darwin's blind process, then everything must be made to fit that story. If, in contrast, you treat the system as designed overall, then you can invoke natural selection where it fits, without any need to force the evidence to fit the theory. For instance, you can use it to "predict" that our ancestors must have had a metabolic system that allowed them to survive and even prosper despite times of food scarcity, since we wouldn't be here otherwise. Then you can go and look for the system.

Darwinism, in contrast, is a Procrustean bed. It requires us to assume that our entire metabolic systems—which can switch between different sources of energy, adjust to different kinds and amounts of food, balance our need to find food with the need to store and conserve energy, and so forth—was an adaptation to *food scarcity*.

Remember, Darwin's mechanism has no foresight. It's blind. It can't think, *Humans will someday spread out across the globe into many different ecosystems, with wildly varying types of food supplies. Let's evolve a complex system to thrive on wildly different diets—from the whale blubber and organ meat diet of the Inuit to the carby tubers of the Kitavans.* No, the mechanism had to cobble together all that flexibility, all that capacity, from our earliest ancestors one tiny glitch at a time, as adaptations to the environment, with no planning ahead for future exigencies. That's because the mechanism can only select for current survival advantage. It can't build a working, interdependent system ahead of time.

Foresight, however, can. And there's the rub. Foresight is the exclusive domain of intelligent agents. Man's capacity to rapidly adapt to different diets has about it, in other words, the look of a plan.

There's no good reason, beyond commitment to the theory, to think that persistent food scarcity gave rise to this integrated and complex system with its myriad feedbacks. This Darwinian answer turns a design problem—*must survive long winters and food shortages*—into its own solution. It's a sleight of hand, not a good explanation.

Sure, Darwinists often imbue "evolution" with the powers of an agent. They'll speak of evolution "choosing" paths, "solving" problems, "searching" spaces, and "building" machines. They'll invoke "evolutionary explanations," when they're just using natural selection to explain some feature of a population. In other cases, they're really sneaking design in. This is no doubt because you can't talk long about living things without invoking design.

Darwin provided materialists with a fig leaf, but we don't need it. Instead, let's simply give natural selection its due without letting it turn into a petty tyrant.

Using Natural Selection to Help Us
Select How and What We Eat

So how can we do that? Again, think of natural selection as a filter across time. If a population has been eating a diet for many hundreds or thousands of years, then that diet has survived a Darwinian winnowing. Therefore, we should give it the benefit of the doubt. It's highly likely that the population is well adapted to the diet, and vice versa. But in the modern age, we've introduced new foods while also finding new ways to keep ourselves from getting weeded out of the gene pool. As a result, there are some things in our diet and environment that have not been sifted by natural selection.

Chief among these are industrial oils from non-fatty seeds such as cotton and soybean; refined sugars; and highly refined grains, none of which have passed this test. They're all of recent vintage, especially in the amounts we consume them. Of course, they don't kill us right off the bat like a big dose of arsenic. We don't have to reject them just because they're new. Still, we should be slow to rely on such untested substances and promote them over natural whole foods that have sustained us for millennia. Add this logic to the pile of evidence we have that the switch was a bad idea.

We should apply the same logic to fasting. Do patterns of fasting and feasting appear in almost every culture for thousands of years—for different reasons? Yes, they do. So we should give the practice the benefit of the doubt—especially since the patterns mimic a much older pattern of periodic food scarcity. Almost all major religions known to history have some fasting tradition. (The one exception is Zoroastrianism, which forbids fasting. How many Zoroastrians have you met lately?) Fasting is not only part of our design plan but has passed through the Darwinian filter. We abandoned it at our own peril.

Does this mean we should find our way back to the hunter-gatherer lifestyle? Should we join Jared Diamond, who wrote famously that "the adoption of agriculture, supposedly our most decisive step toward a better life, was in many ways a catastrophe from which we have never recovered"? Is farming really, as he wrote, "the worst mistake in the history of the human race"?[8] No. That's going too far. True, because we're fallen and finite, we often fail to foresee unintended consequences, and so make a mess of things. Other times, there are real pluses but also some real minuses, with the downside only emerging later. That happens often. Innovation frequently comes with costs that we can't reckon until later. Think of cars, smartphones, and social media. And when we discover such costs, we should do what we can to mitigate them.

At the same time, we don't need to reject innovation and technology, or embrace everything "natural" and reject everything "artificial." After all, the polio virus is natural and the vaccine against it is artificial. Our inventions reflect the fact that we are made in the image of a creative God. They have made it possible for us to be fruitful and multiply and fill the earth and subdue it.

We also shouldn't fall for the opposite error: the transhumanist myth that we will soon merge with our technology and cast off our bodies. There's a middle path of wisdom between these extremes.

We should attend to the wisdom of tradition, to deep ancestral practices, and to the latest evidence from natural science. All three whisper the same message: by abandoning time-honored patterns of feeding, fasting, and feasting with natural foods including natural fats, in favor of grazing on sugar, refined grains, and manufactured fats, we've made ourselves sick, in both body and soul.

When it comes to what and how we eat, it's time to reconnect with our ancestry and our design plan.

Locking In the Fasting Lifestyle

If you make it through our six-week plan, you should have what it takes to make fasting part of your permanent lifestyle. The goal, remember, is to become and remain metabolically flexible. That is, you want to keep your body in a state so that it can burn either sugar or fat, so that it can switch back and forth between these two metabolic pathways. To do this, you need to stay insulin-sensitive and fat-adapted, so your mitochondria stay adept at using fat for fuel.

Okay, you may be thinking, *do I have to stick to a ketogenic diet all the time? Do I have to give up pasta? What about ice cream, beer, Snickers, and brownies?*

The short answer is no. An eat-fast-feast lifestyle need not exclude any foods. Not even birthday cake, donuts, fudge, pumpkin pie, and cannoli. Such treats are among life's pleasures, and I won't tell you to forgo them from now on. The problem is that they are common in our modern lives when they should be reserved for truly special occasions. If you eat someone's birthday cake at your office every week, something's amiss.

Let educated sense and prudence be your guide. That guide

should, however, include most of the following practices. The more of these things you do, the easier it will be to lock in the fasting lifestyle.

1. Don't graze on non-feast days. Make use of regular, time-restricted eating. Jason Fung's single best tip for avoiding obesity is, "Don't eat all the time."[1] The same advice works for fasting. Rarely eat for more than twelve hours in a day and limit your eating window to eight hours whenever you can.

2. Make fasting a part of your daily/weekly/monthly/yearly routine.

3. On regular weeks, keep at least one fast day, but preferably two. To join your efforts with millions of other Christians throughout history, fast on Wednesdays and Fridays. Depending on your needs, you can fast entirely on these days, mimic a fast by consuming only one-fourth of your usual daily calories, or restrict your eating window to one to four hours. If you are overweight, go for more stringent fasts. If you are underweight, be sure to meet your total caloric needs.

4. Anchor your fasting and feasting to the Christian calendar. This will remind you that fasting is a spiritual discipline; unite you in your practice with millions of other Christians; allow you to tap into community support, when many others will also be fasting; and allow you to experience different kinds of fasts over different timescales (more on this later).

5. Mark fast and feast days for the entire year on your calendar. This will make you less dependent on willpower

during weak moments. If an unscheduled birthday party or wedding lands on a day you had marked for a fast, just move the fast up or back one day.

6. Don't go more than a week without entering ketosis. This will keep you metabolically flexible. There are only two ways to do this: fasting and drastic reduction of net carbs, especially high-glycemic ones.

7. Eat modestly on most days. This is much easier to do if you stick with real, lightly processed food.

8. Avoid sugar (including sweet fruit), refined carbs, sweet drinks, and heavily processed food on non-feast days.

9. When carbs are low, increase your consumption of natural fats. Eating fat doesn't mean that your meals will be mostly fat by volume. Fat is calorie dense. The almost invisible olive oil on your salad may have more calories than that six-inch cube of lettuce you've poured it over.

10. Get most of your carbs from green vegetables. In terms of *volume* but not calories, you can follow Michael Pollan's advice, "Eat food, mostly plants, not too much."[2] As much as you can, though, stick with plants that have a very low glycemic load—think spinach not potatoes.

11. Enjoy mini-feasts on Sunday.

12. Enjoy real feast days every so often. (More on this in the next chapter.)

An Example: What I Do

I do all of the above. I've been at this a while and am on the low side of both BMI and body fat. So you might think I could get away with eating a lot of carbs and sweets. But in truth, I eat low-carb or keto most of the time. (That's one of the reasons I have a low BMI and body fat percentage.) I don't eat pasta. Instead, I use spaghetti squash, riced cauliflower, or konjac noodles. I eat precious little bread, white potatoes, or legumes. I never drink fruit juice. Even on rare occasions—such as Thanksgiving—when I eat pie, my wife makes it with almond flour (and Truvía).

I would probably eat this way for improved mental acuity alone. But as we've seen, this eating style has other health benefits as well. I just don't think we're meant to eat much sugar or processed carbohydrates, and I don't see any good reason to regularly eat grains and starches rather than vegetables and nuts.

Last but not least, this way of eating makes it much easier to maintain fasting over the long haul.

You may not want to follow such a strict diet, and so may skip (5) through (7) above. These aren't essential to preserve a fasting lifestyle. We're all unique, with different food preferences and tolerances. I can't eat dairy, eggs, and wheat, for instance, so that limits my options. You may have different issues, or no issues to speak of.

And despite the glycemic index, carbs don't affect everyone the same way. One person may be sensitive to chocolate chip cookies but have no problem with rice. Another person may be fine with the cookies but not the rice. To find out which carbs you tolerate well and which ones do a number on your blood sugar, see the carb test on page 264.

It might not be fair, but some people are naturally lean and insulin sensitive. They can eat gobs of fruits, grains, and starches and do just fine. Others are insulin-resistant and swell up if they even think about a potato. Most of us are somewhere in the middle; though as a population, we're clearly listing toward obesity and insulin resistance.

ROBB WOLF'S SEVEN-DAY CARB TEST[3]

1. Choose a carbohydrate-rich food—apple sauce, chocolate chip cookie, banana, pasta, white rice, white bread, etc.—and measure out fifty grams of effective carbs of this food (that is, total carbs minus fiber.) You'll need to determine how much of the food will get you fifty grams of effective carbs. Do a "food search" for every common food here to get the numbers: https://ndb.nal.usda.gov/ndb/search/list.
2. First thing in the morning, eat your test carb. Don't eat any other food, though you can drink calorie-free coffee, tea, or water. If you drink one of these, make sure to do the same each morning you are testing.
3. Write down the carbohydrate you are testing and when you ate it.
4. Set a timer for two hours.
5. Test your blood glucose and record your blood glucose reading.

For more information, see https://robbwolf.com/wiredtoeat/7daycarbtest/.

Do you have too much body fat? Then a low-carb/low-glycemic load diet combined with the right kinds of fasting might be your best bet for getting rid of the extra blubber and keeping it off. Think meats, natural oils, and lots of green vegetables.

If you've read this far, you already know the reasons why. But here's one more. A large, rigorous 2018 study compared subjects who had recently lost weight after a diet. The subjects eating a low-carb diet for a couple of months burned about 250 calories a day on average more than subjects eating a high-carb diet. That's right. A low-carb or keto diet will probably boost your metabolism. And the more insulin-resistant you are, the greater the effect will be.[4]

Exercise is also important, no matter what body type you have. I work out five to six times a week, for a weekly total of about six hours of vigorous exercise—not counting walking. I do resistance training with weights, with suspension straps, and with bodyweight calisthenics. For cardio, I mostly do HIIT—high-intensity internal training. Aside from the obvious benefits, exercise tends to make us more insulin sensitive, so it's an important part of the fasting lifestyle.

Whatever you do, strive to embed into your life the pattern of eating, fasting, and feasting *at different timescales*. If you do this for several months in a row, you'll be well on your way to locking in this pattern for life.

28

How and Why We Should Feast

If more of us valued food and cheer and song above hoarded
gold, it would be a merrier world.
—Thorin's last words to Bilbo in *The Hobbit* by J. R. R. Tolkien

You may be scratching your head, wondering, Why do we
need a chapter on feasting? After all, by historical standards,
most of us feast every day. And on feast days, we have super-
feasts. At Thanksgiving, we pig out on turkey, dressing, gravy,
mashed potatoes, pumpkin pie, bread pudding, sweet cranberry
dressing, rolls, mounds of butter, and more. Much more. And
then, when we get sleepy, we blame the turkey! It's not the turkey's fault that you're sleepy—that's a myth. It's the crazy infu-
sion of simple carbs. If you put a cubic foot of mashed potatoes
and bready stuffing in your stomach, your body has to process
that, and will have to cut back on resources to your brain that
might have helped you stay awake during the Cowboys game.

But all this eating notwithstanding, we do need to learn how to
feast. Much of what we've been doing isn't really feasting. It's just
eating a lot. A feast is not a free pass to be a drunk and a glutton.

Too often, that's what it has become. Just think of Mardi Gras ("Fat Tuesday"). It started as a final party before the long Lenten fast. Yet how many people, wasted in the streets of Rio de Janeiro and New Orleans, really fast and sacrifice for the next six weeks? A feast, wrenched from its context, tends to descend into debauchery.

Still, if we want to recover a fasting lifestyle, we need to include proper feasts as well. To get our bearings, let's return to Jesus's example.

Jesus Feasted

Jesus fasted for forty days and forty nights before he started his earthly ministry. But in the gospels after that, there's far more feasting than fasting. So much, in fact, that it seemed to cause scandal.

John the Baptist led an austere life in the desert, with his camel-hair tunic and meals of locusts and honey. So did John's disciples. As a result, they were bothered that Jesus's disciples seemed a bit slack.

According to the Gospel of Matthew, John's disciples came to Jesus and asked, "Why do we and the Pharisees fast, but your disciples do not fast?" And Jesus's answer was, "Can the wedding guests mourn as long as the bridegroom is with them? The days will come, when the bridegroom is taken away from them, and then they will fast" (Matt. 19:14–15).

Matthew and Luke report a related comment of Jesus, "For John the Baptist has come eating no bread and drinking no wine; and you say, 'He has a demon.' The Son of man has come eating and drinking; and you say, 'Behold, a glutton and a drunkard, a friend of tax collectors and sinners!' Yet wisdom is justified by all her children" (Luke 7:33–35).

Jesus's point, or at least one of his points, is that there's a time for feasting, and a time for fasting. A wedding is a time for feasting. Jesus's first recorded miracle was the wedding feast at Cana, when he turned big casks of water into wine. The physical presence of Christ, who is the "Bridegroom" of the Church, calls for a wedding feast. In fact, it calls for the mother of all feasts!

The First Christian Feasts

Jesus and his disciples followed the major Jewish feasts. We know from John's gospel that they attended at least three Passovers in Jerusalem during Jesus's earthly ministry. Indeed, the Last Supper that Jesus shared with his disciples before his death was during Passover. And Jesus himself was the sacrificial Lamb, offered in the appearance of bread and wine.

Because Jesus rose from the dead on a Sunday, Christians, from very early on, treated every Sunday as a little feast day when they partook of the Lord's Supper. And it wasn't long before they made the Jewish holy days of Passover (Easter) and Pentecost major *Christian* feasts.

By the fourth century AD, Christians were celebrating Christ's birth (Christmas) and the visit of the wise men (Epiphany). They continued to add more feasts over the centuries—with all manner of days becoming major feasts in some countries.

Before long, the whole calendar was festooned with feast days, so the Church had to prune things back. Many of the minor feasts were either demoted or moved to Sunday—though there is regional variety. For instance, countries and regions often memorialize special saints, either on the anniversary of their birth or death, or on the date of a special apparition or miracle.[1]

Think, for instance, of Mexico and Our Lady of Guadalupe. Or Ireland and St. Patrick.

Rest and Celebrate

Whatever the details, Christians from the beginning have enjoyed feast days/holy days to celebrate what God has done in history. And most still do.

Orthodox Christians have the most intense fasts and the most major feasts. That's no coincidence. For most of history, people didn't have a lot of extra food. To store up extra food for a feast, they had to cut back in the days leading up to it. So the more fasts they had, the more feasts they could enjoy as well.

To speak from my own experience, feasts are a lot more fun and spiritually enriching when they follow a serious fast. A feast is supposed to be a break from work, from fasting, and from our normal routine. A feast is a time of rest—mimicking God's seventh day of the creation week—but it is rest that involves celebration rather than just sleeping late. "Work," Josef Pieper writes in his important study of festivity, "is an everyday occurrence, while a feast is something special, unusual, an interruption in the ordinary passage of time."[2] The English word "leisure" may capture the idea better than the word "rest," since the latter may conjure up images of lying around or sleeping. A feast is a time set aside for leisure and celebration.

Isn't Every Day Holy?

Some Christians object to marking off certain days. After all, isn't every day a free gift of God? Shouldn't we strive for holiness every day, rather than just on "holy days"? Well, yes. Holidays are not excuses to sin on other days. Still, for good reason God *wants us* to set aside special days. Remember, from the beginning, God set aside one day of the week for rest. Was he really tired? Of course not. But his primordial day of "rest" established the model that we are supposed to keep. Perhaps God knows we're creatures of habit who will either work too much or slack off and grow forgetful unless we periodically vary what we do.

God also established special festivals, with specific rules and rubrics, that observant Jews keep to this day. A day of rest, and special days of celebration, weren't supposed to come to an end when Christ ascended into heaven. Christ did not come to abolish this pattern of work, fast, rest, feast, but to fulfill it.

"'A holiday every day'—even every other day—is an idea that cannot be realized in practice," writes Josef Pieper. "A festival can arise only out of a foundation of a life whose ordinary shape is given by the working day." Without meaningful work, the whole thing falls apart: "An idle-rich class of do-nothings," he notes wryly, "are hard put even to amuse themselves, let alone to celebrate a festival."[3] Fasts and feasts cast light on each other, and on ordinary days. And those ordinary days help give meaning to the fasts and the feasts.

Wait, Isn't That a Sin?

Some of us might have another lingering worry: Should you *enjoy* the revelry of any feast, since the world and our bodies are so mired in sin? Aren't big feasts and parties, with their eating and drinking and—gasp!—dancing, too spiritually dangerous to trifle with? Perhaps the best we can do is to strive every day to detach ourselves from such bodily pleasures and to await the Kingdom to come.

Of course, few Christians follow this logic to its bitter end. To see it reduced to the absurd, consider one of those seventeenth-century portraits of a Puritan clad in black, sporting a stiff white collar that looks like a compressed accordion. He looks as if his face would crumble if he cracked a smile. He prizes not just sobriety but also cheerlessness. Did you know that for a few years in the 1600s, public Christmas celebrations were *prohibited by law* in England? Puritans in Massachusetts even forbade Christmas merriment from 1659 to 1681.[4]

Clearly, these folks had settled on a half-truth. (Catholics had their own version, called Jansenism.) Yes, we should seek to detach ourselves from worldly affections—that's one of the reasons we should fast. Many people do like to binge on fine food and fine wine. But it doesn't follow that we should never celebrate what God has done. On the contrary! We should seek to remind ourselves that this is God's world. Yes, it's fallen, but it is still good. It's not just *okay* to celebrate God's world and his works. We *should* do so.

Not a "Cheat Day"

But have you met any Puritans (or Jansenists) lately? Probably not. Puritanism is a less common impulse now than it was a few centuries ago. Still, vestiges of it linger on if we treat feasts as "cheat days"—that is, as departures from how we really should be eating. If you've spent years going on and off of diets, and are just now learning how to fast, you'll need to guard against this error. So, repeat after me: *Feast days are not cheat days. Feast days are not cheat days. Feast days are not cheat days.*

Why? Well, first, the idea of a cheat day doesn't make sense. To cheat is to deceive or trick someone. If you make cheat notes for a test, you're deceiving your teacher. But if you decide to set aside a day to eat something you generally avoid, whom have you deceived?[5] No one. You've just set dietary limits and chosen to make exceptions on certain days, perhaps in hope that the weekly donut and pasta spree will keep you on track on the other days.

Second, feast days are not days set aside to eat something you shouldn't. They're not exceptions to the more proper way of acting. They are an essential part of the whole. More than that, they are a summit and goal of the pattern of eating, fasting, and feasting. I've used the shorthand term "fasting lifestyle," but feasts are as much a part of the story as are the fasts.

Nutritionism

Nowadays, the subtlest form of puritanism is to treat food and drink as nothing but fuel. If you're really into fitness or dieting, you should watch out for this error.

We've had to talk about macro- and micronutrients in this book in order to grasp how our diet has changed recently, and what this change has done to our metabolism. We've spent decades restricting natural fats and boosting our intake of sugar and refined carbs, and we needed to take some time to dismantle this misguided mental food pyramid. When all is said and done, however, we should think in terms of whole foods, not abstract parts. Food is far more than fuel.

You don't directly encounter calories, carbohydrates, fats, and proteins. Even at the level of chemistry, real foods have far more to them. We may think of a chicken breast as just a source of protein. In truth, it's a complex matrix of hundreds of different elements and compounds, of proteins and fats, of the history of a specific chicken—a history it retains even when it is grilled and served to us with broccoli and cauliflower.

Eating isolated chicken protein, or amino acids from such protein, is not the same thing as eating an actual chicken breast. Taking a vitamin C tablet is not the same thing as getting vitamin C from a grapefruit. Our bodies are designed to make use of grapefruit. Vitamin tablets are recent additions.

We eat T-bones, cherries, guacamole, chocolate cinnamon cake, hummus, olive oil, and sourdough bread—all of which are far more complex than their energy content and their macronutrient and micronutrient profile. A lipid scientist could bore you to tears describing the intricacies of humble olive oil.

Treating food as nothing but fuel is a uniquely modern error. It's a type of reductionism that had very bad effects in the twentieth century. Once scientists could isolate the energy content of food, it led them to fixate on macronutrients (recall that fat has nine calories per gram, protein and carbohydrates each has four). Isolating micronutrients such as vitamins and minerals had much the same effect. These discoveries fed the temptation to focus on what we can measure—fat, calories, total cholesterol—and to ignore or dismiss what we can't.

Michael Pollan calls this modern trend *nutritionism*.[6] It happens when we focus on isolated ingredients rather than whole foods in their complex natural forms and cultural settings. Yes, we can and should be aware of the nutrition content of the foods we eat. But if we are to enjoy feasts, we need to avoid nutritionism.

Feasting Together

Imagine a seventy-year-old woman named Betty. She gets up early on Christmas morning, stuffs a turkey with corn-bread dressing and puts it in the oven. She makes sweet potato casserole and green bean casserole, cranberry salad, and pumpkin pie. She mixes eggnog using an old family recipe. She boils mulled wine on the stove, makes chocolate fudge, and sets out a pecan-dense fruit cake she got from a niece in Texas. She lays out a red tablecloth on her long dining room table. On top, she places an Advent wreath, her finest Christmas china—Lenox Holiday Tartan—red crystal goblets, and the antique sterling silver flatware she hardly every uses. She lights all the candles on the wreath and turns on her favorite Christmas music—Lessons and Carols from the King's College Boys Choir. Then she sits down, says grace, and eats . . . alone.

Depressing image, isn't it? I can barely stand to think about it. Feasts are meant to be enjoyed with others—usually with our closest family members and close friends. A feast enjoyed alone is less a feast than a symbol of loneliness and isolation. We react viscerally to the thought of someone spending Thanksgiving or Christmas or Easter alone. As we should. We are social beings. No woman gives birth to herself. No man is an island. We are (ideally) born into families. We live in neighborhoods nestled in cities, located within countries. One of the first things God says in the Bible is, "It is not good that man should be alone" (Gen. 2:18). We know from scientific studies (as if we needed them) that our social ties are one of the key ingredients for long-term happiness. Loneliness doesn't just make us sad. It can make us sick.

Though there are many communal fasts, it's possible to fast alone. Feasts, in contrast, are inherently social. That's why, on major holidays, we feel the absence of family members more acutely. These events are meant to bring us together and to be enjoyed together.

All Together Now

Even when we're eating alone, we don't normally consume whole foods in isolation. Unlike animals, which eat their food raw off the ground, we prepare, cook, and eat food while sitting upright at tables. These foods are usually transformed in recipes and even cuisines, which are themselves far richer and more complex than the individual foods they contain. Cuisines, almost always enhanced with spices and special styles of cooking, are products of places, climates, people groups, and histories. They resonate with a past that might otherwise be long forgotten. They remind us of those who have gone before.

We have special foods anchored in cultural and religious traditions that may date back centuries or even millennia. These "pleasures of the table" separate us from other animals, for which the enjoyment of eating is just biological.[7] No chimpanzee ever prayed before eating or proposed a toast or baked a wedding cake.

This cultural dimension is especially true of foods and dishes we eat during feasts. How often do you eat turkey and dressing in months other than November and December? What about pumpkin pie, or eggnog, or cranberry dressing? And food is only part of the picture. We elaborate feasts with special decorations and table wear. We sing songs, watch and march in parades, decorate with special plants and flowers, put trees up in our living room, and wear special clothing. We may even don garish sweaters that we pull out once a year.

At Christmas, we exchange gifts. At Easter, we exchange candy and dye boiled eggs and buy new dress clothes. At Thanksgiving? Well, we give thanks and eat a lot. That's fitting. This national holiday was established to enjoy with gratitude the bounty that God has blessed us with as Americans.

These festivities serve to remind us of, and re-present to us, the great things God has done in history and in our lives. Don't feel naughty or squeamish about enjoying feasts. On the contrary. Throw yourself into them with gusto! For it is to a feast that all of our fasting ultimately points.

Conclusion: From the Primordial Fast to the Wedding Feast of the Lamb

The proper pattern of Christian eating, fasting, and feasting is like a fractal. A fractal is a geometric figure that is rendered by a simple algorithm and that maintains the same coherent structure at every size scale. This property distinguishes a fractal from other shapes. If you look at, say, one edge of a large black circle on your computer screen, and slowly zoom in, the circle will pass out of view, the line will get thicker and thicker, more and more pixelated, and before long it won't look like anything. Just a black screen.

In contrast, when you watch a fractal—such as the famous Mandelbrot Set—scale up or down on a screen, you see mesmerizing patterns continue like a fractured coastline that just keeps fracturing—forever. The fractures aren't random but recur in beautiful patterns. If you don't know what I'm talking about, pause for a minute, go online and find a video of the "Mandelbrot fractal zoom" and run it. It's easier to experience than to describe in words. The figure on page 278 is only one still shot of the Mandelbrot Set as it appears at a certain resolution on a computer screen or printed page.

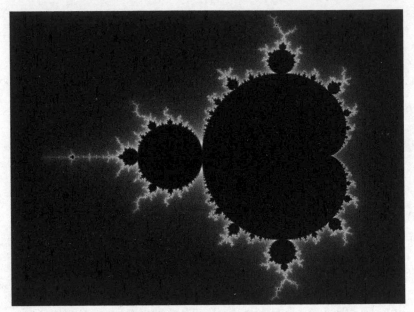

Two-dimensional still of the Mandelbrot Set at one resolution, created by Wolfgang Beyer with *Ultrafractal 3*, Wikimedia Commons, grayscale

Some have called fractals the "fingerprints of God." They recur not just on 2-D computer screens (where we can behold their wonders), but in the shapes of mountains, trees and other plants, hurricanes, galaxies, nautilus and other seashells— even clouds, which until recently looked to most people like random shapes. In fact, the shapes of clouds are highly ordered, not random. Fractals are God's little Easter eggs hidden in his creation.

It's fitting, then, that our short lives on earth should conform to a fractal pattern across time.

We have the daily pattern of times when we eat and work. This pattern is repeated at much smaller, faster scales, in our

cells, our mitochondria, and our gut microbes. We have the recurring day and night of every twenty-four-hour day. We eat
during the daytime and fast at night—just as God created from
morning to evening during his creation week and rested from
evening to morning. When we fix this pattern in our daily and
weekly lives, we imitate a pattern established by God himself.

For many centuries, Christians marked every week with a
similar pattern—fasting on Wednesday and Friday and celebrating a small feast on Sunday.

With Ember Days, they marked the four seasons of the year,
the times of sowing and reaping, planting and harvesting. This
is the only place where the Christian calendar has taken its cue
from the annual changes in climate. Otherwise, the crests and
troughs of the Christian year are defined by two great moments
of Christian history: when God came to Earth as a child born to
a young virgin, and when he rose from the dead as a first fruit of
the eternal—bodily—life to come. To mark these moments, we
have great feasts preceded by two longs seasons of fasting.

Altogether, this provides both repetition and change—theme
and variation—just as one expects to see in great art and music.[1]
Enough pattern and routine to form habits. Enough variation to
prevent plateaus and mindless repetition.

For instance, the Ember Days come at the beginning of each
of the four seasons, and always land on Wednesday, Friday, and
Saturday. (And if you match food to seasons, as most people did
for most of history, then you'll even eat some different foods
around each of the four fasts.) These fasts break up our weekly
eating pattern, but not randomly.

Then there are the special fasts and feasts of Advent/Christmas
and Lent/Easter. While Christmas Day wanders around the days

of the week, it lands on the same calendar date. So it's an "immovable feast." In contrast, Lent and Easter are "movable feasts": because they're tied to the lunar calendar, they always land on the same days of the week—Ash Wednesday, Easter Sunday, and so forth—but wander around the annual calendar by as much as a month.

Various other feast days pepper the annual calendar. Some are more or less universal. Others are specific to countries, parishes, and religious orders.

National holidays add more variation. In the United States, for instance, Independence Day always lands on July 4, whereas Thanksgiving—our biggest national feast—lands on the fourth Thursday of November—whatever the date.

The result is that we never fully settle into a simple monotonous pattern, which our minds and metabolisms can automate. But neither are we adrift in a sea of random events. Such a complex but non-random pattern is perfect for bodily creatures of both habit, which can become automatic, and the capacity for virtue, which requires conscious effort.

Even over the course of our lives, there are times when we predominately feed—infancy—and times when we predominantly fast—as we near death.

I suspect that this pattern of different timescales has both spiritual and physical benefits. And different fasts have different effects. Longer nighttime fasting may be associated with reduced breast cancer risk, for instance. And, within reason, the longer the fast, the stronger the effect.[2]

For just bringing down insulin, burning fat, and boosting growth hormone, eighteen to twenty-four hours seems to be the sweet spot.[3] For autophagy, we need to fast for a longer period. It may be that for fighting some diseases—such as cancer—longer fasts, whether water-only or mimicking, will be called for.

The Wedding Feast of the Lamb

What about spiritual benefits? If you think (as I do) that the Holy Spirit guides and protects the Church, then you might suspect that there is wisdom in traditional Christian practice beyond what we can discover in a clinical trial. We should, at least, give that practice the benefit of the doubt, especially since it seems to foreshadow life in the Kingdom of God.

The Church Fathers noticed that the Bible, and human history, begins with a fast and ends with a feast. Early in Genesis, God tells Adam and Eve that they may enjoy any of the fruits of the garden but for the fruit from one tree. If we remember that first fast, which our first parents failed to keep, how much more glorious is the feast at the end of Scripture when time itself is fulfilled.

But how does our fasting and feasting in this life relate to the wedding feast that John describes in Revelation? On the one hand, because of sin, neither our world nor our bodies are the way they're supposed to be. On the other hand, it is God's world and he will bring it to fruition in his own time. And when he does, it will not be a ghostly existence with our souls floating around on clouds. We believe not just in eternal life, but in the resurrection of the body, in a new heaven and a new earth (Rev. 21).

Mysteriously, Jesus ate fish with his disciples after his resurrection. And it is through a form of eating that he makes his saving work available to us. He came in the flesh, and offered his flesh to save us, body and soul. "I am the living bread which came down from heaven," he said; "if any one eats of this bread, he will live for ever; and the bread which I shall give for the life of the world is my flesh" (John 6:51).

The disciples were accustomed to Jesus speaking with parables and metaphors. When his disciples heard Jesus speak these words, however, they didn't translate it into metaphor in their heads. They balked. And Jesus didn't respond by clearing up any misunderstanding. Nor did John explain to readers that the Lord was just using a figure of speech. John reports instead that Jesus pressed the point:

> *Truly, truly, I say to you, unless you eat the flesh of the Son of man and drink his blood, you have no life in you; he who eats my flesh and drinks my blood has eternal life, and I will raise him up at the last day. For my flesh is food indeed, and my blood is drink indeed (John 6:53–55).*

The word John uses for "eat" here is better translated "chew." It foreshadows Jesus's command at the Last Supper, which is described in the other three gospels. Jesus held bread and told his gathered disciples, "Take, eat; this is my body." Then, "he took a cup, and when he had given thanks he gave it to them, saying, 'Drink of it, all of you; for this is my blood of the covenant, which is poured out for many for the forgiveness of sins'" (Matt. 26:26–28). He didn't say abstractly, "I am the bread" or "I am the cup." He said, rather, "this is my body" and "this is my blood." It's as if, rather than saying, "I am the door," Jesus had pointed to one particular door and said, "See this door right here? *This* door is my body. You have to walk through it to achieve eternal life."

The hardness of the saying about chewing flesh and drinking blood was not lost on its original audience. John tells us that as a result of Jesus's statement, "many of his disciples drew back and no longer went about with him" (John 6:66). Jesus did not call them back. Peter and the rest of the twelve remained, steadfast but bewildered. As did the millions of Christians who followed them down the centuries.

These days, we're tempted to explain these words away or to look past them without really reading them. We want to "spiritualize" this fleshly message of eating and drinking a sacrificial offering. *Of eating Jesus's body and drinking his blood.* In a similar way, we may imagine that our bodily existence is temporary, that our salvation, and the way God chose to gain it for us, is not so much about our bodies as our souls.

But if we accept what Jesus says realistically,[4] then we can see more clearly how our fasting and feasting anticipate the kingdom of God. Especially in the Eucharist, they provide us with constant reminders that the unity of body and soul will not be left behind but will be taken up and transformed in the life to come (1 Cor. 15:44). The incarnation is about God becoming flesh and saving us in the flesh with his flesh. We are unities of heaven and earth, of the dust of the ground and the breath of God. As a result, our bodies are not mere physical objects independent of the spiritual realm but vessels through which God chooses to raise us to himself. "The body alone," notes St. Pope John Paul II, "is capable of making visible what is invisible: the spiritual and the divine. It was created to transfer into the visible reality of the world, the mystery hidden since time immemorial in God, and thus to be a sign of it."[5]

What will it be like to live with God in a glorified body? How should we imagine an eternal wedding *feast*? We should not picture it as static and lifeless. What if you never needed to rest, or eat, or sleep, or exercise? You would never have the desire to eat or drink, never really enjoy a good meal. If you never felt tired, you could never enjoy a good night's sleep. How much richer is an earthly life punctuated by patterns of work and rest, of fasts and feasts.

Perhaps this pattern also gives us a glimpse of the eternal—embodied—lives of the blessed. We will not be at risk of starvation of course. But life in the kingdom of God will surely not be, as Arnold Toynbee said about history, "just one damned thing after the other." Nor will it leave our existence an "undistinguishable heap," as Shelley complained of Christianity.[6] It will not be like an earthly meal where we have to keep eating and eating, even after our stomachs are distended. It surely will offer theme and variation, contrast, joys, and surprises without end. Like the inexhaustible God himself, it will be ever ancient and ever new.

As John Piper says in *A Hunger for God*:

> One might think that those who feast most often on communion with God are least hungry. . . . But, paradoxically, it is not so that they are the least hungry saints. . . . The strongest, most mature Christians I have ever met are the hungriest for God. It might seem that those who eat most would be least hungry. But that's not the way it works with an inexhaustible fountain, and an infinite feast, and a glorious Lord.[7]

The Church Fathers made much of the parallels between the Eucharist and the eschatological vision of John in the book of Revelation. Indeed, they saw John's vision as in part a

description, from the heavenly vantage point, of what is happening even now in the Lord's Supper, when heaven comes to
earth. (Scott Hahn's delightful book *The Lamb's Supper* gives a
great summary of these insights.)[8] Just as Jews during Passover
must eat the lamb in order to have God's forgiveness applied to
them, so too do we feast on the Lamb slain once for all in time,
and in eternity (Heb. 7:27; Rev. 13:8)—though it is a Lamb
hidden under the appearance of an offering of bread and wine.

In the Wedding Feast of the Lamb, John heaps symbol
upon symbol. The "Lion of the tribe of Judah" who conquers
evil and death is also a "Lamb, standing as though it had been
slain" (Rev. 5:5–6)—a most unlikely image of a cosmic victor.
That same Lamb is also Host and Bridegroom of a wedding feast
with the Church as the Bride. The Lamb is the Sacrificial Offering and also the Wedding Feast (Rev. 19:6–9). Later in the text,
John describes the Lamb as both the Temple and its Lamp! He is
stretching to describe realities beyond our current imaginings,
and seems to be saying, "Don't even try to picture this."

What is clear is that the Lamb's Feast refers to the con-
summation of all things in the Kingdom of God, in a new
Jerusalem, a new heaven, and a new earth, when Satan and
death are finally vanquished. It reminds us, one last time, that
we are now, and ever shall be, *bodily* beings. In our eating,
our fasting, and our feasting, then, we have a foretaste of that
great feast to come—when, in our glorified bodies, we will see,
know, love, glorify, and enjoy God forever.

ACKNOWLEDGMENTS

Thanks to Jonathan Witt, who read much of the manuscript and offered characteristically valuable edits. I'd also like to thank Anika Smith, Kathleen Abela, and my wife, Ginny Richards, who offered me valuable feedback on the multi-week plan laid out in the book. Ginny also read the manuscript in its entirety and suggested a number of improvements.

Thanks to Mickey Maudlin of HarperOne as well as my agent Giles Anderson, who have made this the smoothest and most pain-free book project in my experience.

This book exists in large part because of people who have read articles I've written on fasting, or heard me speak about fasting, and encouraged me to combine my reflections on the subject into a book. Thanks to all of you for this crowdsourced advice. I took it as a sign that I should write the book.

APPENDIX 1. ADDITIONAL BOOKS

Maria Augusta von Trapp, *Around the Year with the Von Trapp Family*

Thomas Dubay, *Deep Conversion, Deep Prayer*

——, *Fire Within: St. Theresa of Avila, St. John of the Cross, and the Gospel—On Prayer*

Jason Fung, *The Diabetes Code: Prevent and Reverse Type 2 Diabetes Naturally*

——, *The Obesity Code: Unlocking the Secrets of Weight Loss*

Bobby Gross, *Living the Christian Year: Time to Inhabit the Story of God*

Scott Hahn, *The Lamb's Supper: The Mass as Heaven on Earth*

St. John Paul II, *Salvifici Doloris*

Leon Kass, *The Hungry Soul: Eating and the Perfecting of Our Nature*

Ralph Martin, *The Fulfillment of All Desire: A Guidebook for the Journey to God Based on the Wisdom of the Saints*

Josef Pieper, *In Tune with the World: A Theory of Festivity*

Gary Taubes, *The Case Against Sugar*

——, *Good Calories, Bad Calories: Fats, Carbs, and the Controversial Science of Diet and Health*

——, *Why We Get Fat: And What to Do About It*

Nina Teicholz, *The Big Fat Surprise: Why Butter, Meat, and Cheese Belong in a Healthy Diet*

Kendra Tierney, *The Catholic All Year Compendium: Liturgical Living for Real Life*

Jeff Volek and Stephen Phinney, *The Art and Science of Low Carbohydrate Living*

Dallas Willard, *The Spirit of the Disciplines: Understanding How God Changes Lives*

Robb Wolf, *Wired to Eat: Turn Off Cravings, Rewire Your Appetite for Weight Loss, and Determine the Foods That Work for You*

Martha Zimmerman, *Celebrating the Christian Year*

Week One

Eat a "ketogenic" diet of high natural fat, moderate protein, and very low carbs (below fifty grams not counting fiber) without simple sugars, grains, or starches. Get about 80 percent of your calories from fat, 15 percent from protein, and 5 percent from carbohydrates. Think natural fats—such as olive and coconut oil—and fatty meats. For carbs, focus on green vegetables grown above ground—such as spinach, broccoli, and asparagus. This way of eating allows your body to shift to a state of "ketosis," in which it draws most of its energy from dietary and body fat. Drink lots of water and increase your salt intake.

Have a mini-feast on Sunday: Enjoy a piece of fruit or some 85 percent dark chocolate.

Week Two

Start to restrict your feeding window to 16/8. That is, every day, fast for sixteen hours (including your night's sleep) and eat all your daily calories (mostly fat, protein, and vegetables) during an eight-hour feeding window.

Have a mini-feast on Sunday and expand your eating window to twelve hours.

Week Three

Lengthen your daily fast with a 20/4 routine. That is, eat all your meals within a four-hour window of time during the day. You don't need to try to restrict calories. This way of eating helps break the habit of eating at fixed times and amplifies the good effects of the ketogenic diet.

Then, on Sunday, have another mini-feast.

Week Four

For three days this week—preferably Monday, Wednesday, and Friday—eat all your food during a one-hour window. You still don't need to try to restrict net calories. Maintain a time-restricted ketogenic diet on other days.

And enjoy a mini-feast on Sunday.

Week Five

Mimic a real fast on Monday, Wednesday, and Friday. Consume one-fourth the number of calories that you normally do—five hundred to six hundred calories. (Think two avocados with lime juice and salt.) Continue with a regular, time-restricted ketogenic diet on the other days.

Plus another mini-feast day on Sunday.

Week Six

For the first few days of the week, prepare for a fast longer than twenty-four hours. Shoot for thirty-six to seventy-two hours. Then sometime on Wednesday through Saturday, observe your fast. By this time, you should be "fat-adapted" and much more metabolically flexible. You'll have felt the benefits of fasting.

Enjoy a proper feast on Sunday.

If you're like me, you'll want to confirm that the strategy is working—that you really are switching your body into fat-burning mode. It would be nice to measure insulin directly, but that's hard and expensive. Second best is to measure whether your blood sugar is staying on the low side of normal and your body is converting fat to ketones and burning them for fuel. The good news is that there are some inexpensive ways to do both.

Urine Strips

The easiest and cheapest tool to test for ketones is a urine strip. A box of 150 strips costs no more than ten dollars. You just pee in a cup, dip the business side of the strip in your urine, pull it out, wait forty seconds, and look at the color change.

If the tip stays tan, that means you're excreting hardly any ketones. Light pink means there are trace amounts. Mauve to purple means there are plenty of ketones in your urine.

If you've just been at this for a few weeks and are following the protocols, the strip should change color. But this method has its limits. The strips detect only one of the three ketones your body produces, called acetoacetate. And it doesn't detect the ones you're *using*, but rather the ones that you're *excreting* through your urine.

As your body becomes more "keto-adapted," it gets better at using ketones for fuel. That means that the urine strips will show fewer and fewer ketones the longer you eat a ketogenic diet. I've been at this for a while, and even when I know I'm in ketosis, the urine strips don't change color for me. To see what's happening for the first month or so, however, urine ketone strips are still the easiest choice.

Blood Tests

If you want to detect ketones and glucose in your blood, you'll need to get a blood testing meter. There are several on the market, but I use the DSS Precision Xtra by Abbott. The kit comes with a digital detector and a little thingy called a "lancet device" that you use to prick your finger. You just pull back a knob, put the other end on the tip of a finger, and push the button. Don't worry. It makes only a tiny prick, enough to render one drop of blood.

You'll also need to buy glucose test strips and ketone test strips. If you buy the meter kit, plus thirty glucose and thirty ketone strips, it will cost you about a hundred dollars. Shop and compare prices on Amazon or other online stores to find the best deals. Buying the strips in bulk will save you money.

Costs would get out of hand quickly if you did these tests every day, since the ketone strips cost over a dollar a piece.

But there's no need to do the test that often. For now, you just want to know if you're producing ketones and lowering your blood sugar.

I recommend doing the same test every few days, or once a week, at a fixed time. Just remember to compare apples with apples. Blood ketones and glucose go up and down throughout the day. Don't compare a test you took right after you had a giant meal at 7:00 p.m., with a test you took first thing in the morning on an empty stomach. Be systematic and write down the numbers.

The blood ketone test tells you the concentration of beta-hydroxybutyrate (BHB) in your blood. That's the ketone your brain really likes to run on.

So, What Should I Look For?

If you're in ketosis, the meter should give you a reading of at least 0.5 mmol/L. (Don't worry about the units. Just look at the number.)

Ideally, you'd like to see it between one and three mmol/L sometime during the day. This is the range that low-carb researchers Jeff Volek and Stephen Phinney call nutritional ketosis.[1]

If you take the test at different times and get readings larger than one, you're fine. If you never get a reading of even 0.5, that means you're not getting into ketosis. The likely culprits? Too many carbs, and maybe too much protein.[2] You may be insulin resistant. In that case, you'll need to drop your daily net carbs to under thirty or even twenty grams a day to kickstart your fat-burning system. Everyone is different. Just keep tweaking your intake of carbs and protein until you hit the sweet spot.

The "normal" blood sugar range for non-diabetics is from seventy to one hundred mg/dL. It will be on the lower end of that range when you're fasting, and on the higher end after you've had a meal. (My fasting blood glucose is around seventy, lower if I'm in nutritional ketosis.) The main thing to check for now is whether both your fasted and fed glucose levels go down as you become more keto-adapted and fit for fasting. Assuming you're otherwise healthy, the trend, not isolated numbers, is what you want to watch.

If you're healthy and you've been on a ketogenic diet for a couple of months, your blood sugar may go well below the normal range. Mine often does. If a doctor were to test my fasting blood sugar when I'm in ketosis, he might think I'm dangerously hypoglycemic, and wonder why I'm not lightheaded. But a lower blood sugar is okay as long as your body is using ketones for fuel.

Things can get more complicated long term[3] when blood sugar can be higher in the morning than you might expect, but don't worry about that now. Just stick with the basics. (If you really want to dive into the details, see the link in this endnote.)[4] Ideally, you will enter ketosis before the end of the first week. So it's helpful to verify that this is happening.

NOTES

INTRODUCTION

1. For the background on the pyramid, see "Food Guide Pyramid," USDA Center for Nutrition Policy and Promotion, at https://www.cnpp.usda.gov/FGP.
2. See it at https://www.choosemyplate.gov/.
3. S. O'Neill and L. O'Driscoll, "Metabolic Syndrome: A Closer Look at a Growing Epidemic and Its Associated Pathology," *Obesity Review* 16, no. 1 (2015): 112.
4. Francesca Bacardi, "Twitter CEO Jack Dorsey Eats Only One Meal per Day," *Page Six*, April 11, 2019, https://pagesix.com/2019/04/11/twitter-ceo-jack-dorsey-eats-only-one-meal-per-day/.
5. Charles Murphy, *The Spirituality of Fasting: Rediscovering a Christian Practice* (Notre Dame, IN: Ave Maria Press, 2010), ix.
6. See the discussion and links at Jimmy Moore, "Can a Christian Follow a Paleo and Low-Carb Diet?" *Livin' La Vida Low Carb*, November 7, 2010, http://livinlavidalowcarb.com/blog/can-a-christian-follow-a-paleo-low-carb-diet/9381.
7. Indeed, even apart from the way we process it, we have radically modified wheat, especially in the last half century. Some argue that this has led to all manner of food sensitivities and illness. See, for example, William Davis, *Wheat Belly: Lose the Weight, Lose the Wheat, and Find Your Way Back to Health* (New York: Rodale Books, 2011).

CHAPTER 1

1. J. D. O'Neill, "Fast," *The Catholic Encyclopedia* (New York: Robert Appleton Company, 1909), http://www.newadvent.org/cathen/05789c.htm.
2. In his first sermon *About Fasting*, 1.3, at https://bible.org/seriespage/appendix-1-basil%E2%80%99s-sermons-about-fasting.
3. Augustine, "On Prayer and Fasting" (LXXII).

4. Neel Burton, "The Extraordinary Life of St. Anthony of the Desert," *Psychology Today*, April 12, 2012, updated September 6, 2017, https://www.psychologytoday.com/us/blog/hide-and-seek/201204/the-extraordinary-life-st-anthony-the-desert.
5. "Anthony of Egypt," *Christianity Today*, https://www.christianitytoday.com/history/people/innertravelers/antony-of-egypt.html.
6. Mark Galli, "Anthony and the Desert Fathers: From the Editors—Models or Kooks?" *Christian History* 69 (1999).
7. Gregory Dix, *The Shape of the Liturgy* (London: Dacre, 1943), 354–55.
8. Charles Murphy, *The Spirituality of Fasting: Rediscovering a Christian Practice* (Notre Dame, IN: Ave Maria Press, 2010), 17.
9. See for instance this inspiring story of Brother Yun by Hui Li Chan at *Inspirational Christians*, http://www.inspirationalchristians.org/biography/brother-yun/.

CHAPTER 2

1. Charles Murphy, *The Spirituality of Fasting: Rediscovering a Christian Practice* (Notre Dame, IN: Ave Maria Press, 2010), 1.
2. Kent Berghuis, *Christian Fasting: A Theological Approach* (Biblical Studies Press, 2007), 119ff.
3. Richard J. Janet, "The Decline of General Fasts in Victorian England, 1832–1857" (dissertation, University of Notre Dame, 1984), 3.
4. Richard Foster, *Celebration of Discipline: The Path to Spiritual Growth* (San Francisco: HarperSanFrancisco, 1988, rev. ed.), 47.
5. J. D. O'Neill, "The Black Fast," *The Catholic Encyclopedia* (New York: Robert Appleton Company, 1907), http://www.newadvent.org/cathen/02590c.htm.
6. J. D. O'Neill, "Fast," *The Catholic Encyclopedia*, http://www.newadvent.org/cathen/05789c.htm.
7. Deacon Joseph Suaiden, "How Did Catholic Fasting Rules Change Throughout History?" *Quora*, February 20, 2015, https://www.quora.com/how-did-catholic-fasting-rules-change-throughout-history#.
8. "Meat" doesn't include reptiles and amphibians either. So, strictly speaking, Catholics can eat salamanders and iguanas on Fridays during Lent. This fact matters to almost no one.
9. Suaiden, 21.
10. Code of Canon Law, http://www.vatican.va/archive/ENG1104/P4O.htm.
11. Elizabeth Scalia, "Common Penance: Why Not Restore Meatless Fridays for the US Church?" *Word on Fire*, August 30, 2018, https://

www.wordonfire.org/resources/blog/common-penance-why-not
-restore-meatless-fridays-for-the-us-church/5888/.

CHAPTER 3

1. See the review essay on the evidence from studies of modern hunter-gatherers, as well as archaeological evidence, in Ann Gibbons, "The Evolution of Diet," *National Geographic*, https://www.national geographic.com/foodfeatures/evolution-of-diet/.

2. On the other hand, there are animal sources of vitamin C, and people who live on an all-meat diet may not need as much vitamin C as the rest of us.

3. Tanya Lewis, "Here's What Fruits and Vegetables Looked Like Before We Domesticated Them," *Business Insider*, January 31, 2016, https://www.businessinsider.com/what-foods-looked-like-before-genetic -modification-2016-1/.

4. James Kennedy, "Artificial vs. Natural Watermelon & Sweetcorn," *James Kennedy*, July 14, 2014, https://jameskennedymonash.wordpress .com/2014/07/14/artificial-vs-natural-watermelon-sweetcorn/.

5. Kennedy, "Artificial vs. Natural Watermelon & Sweetcorn."

6. Rachel K. Johnson, Lawrence J. Appel, Michael Brands, Barbara V. Howard, Michael Lefevre, Robert H. Lustig, Frank Sacks, Lyn M. Steffen, Judith Wylie-Rosett, "Dietary Sugars Intake and Cardiovascular Health: A Scientific Statement from the American Heart Association," *Circulation* 120, no. 11 (September 15, 2009): 1011–20.

7. See chart and references in Kris Gunnar, "11 Graphs That Show Everything That Is Wrong with the Modern Diet," *Healthline*, June 8, 2017, https://www.healthline.com/nutrition/11-graphs-that-show -what-is-wrong-with-modern-diet.

8. Adda Bjarnadottir, "Why Refined Carbs Are Bad for You," *Healthline*, June 4, 2017, https://www.healthline.com/nutrition/why-refined -carbs-are-bad.

9. http://sugarscience.ucsf.edu/hidden-in-plain-sight/#.W41q15NKg6h.

CHAPTER 4

1. A. Keys, J. Brozek, A. Henschel, O. Mickelson, and H. L. Taylor, *The Biology of Human Starvation*, vols. 1–2 (Minneapolis, MN: University of Minnesota Press, 1950).

2. David Baker and Natacha Keramidas, "The Psychology of Hunger," *Psychology Today* 44, no. 9 (October 2013), http://www.apa.org /monitor/2013/10/hunger.aspx.

3. Art Markman, "It Matters Whether You Believe in Willpower," *Psychology Today*, December 10, 2010, https://www.psychologytoday .com/us/blog/ulterior-motives/201012/it-matters-whether-you-believe -in-willpower.

4. Brenda Goodman, "How Your Appetite Can Sabotage Your Weight Loss," *WebMD*, October 14, 2016, https://www.webmd.com/diet /news/20161014/how-your-appetite-can-sabotage-weight-loss#1.

5. Harriet Brown, "The Weight of the Evidence," *Slate*, March 24, 2015, http://www.slate.com/articles/health_and_science/medical _examiner/2015/03/diets_do_not_work_the_thin_evidence_that _losing_weight_makes_you_healthier.html.

6. C. Zauner, B. Schneeweiss, A. Kranz, C. Madl, K. Ratheiser, L. Kramer, E. Roth, B. Schneider, and K. Lenz, "Resting Energy Expenditure in Short-Term Starvation Is Increased as a Result of an Increase in Serum Norepinephrine," *American Journal of Clinical Nutrition* 71, no. 6 (June 2000): 1511–15.

7. Lyle McDonald, "The 3500 Calorie Rule," *Bodyrecomposition*, August 5, 2015, https://bodyrecomposition.com/fat-loss/3500-calorie-rule .html/.

8. Jason Fung, "Fasting Myths—Part 5," *Intensive Dietary Management*, https://idmprogram.com/fasting-myths-part-5/.

9. Jason Fung, "Fasting and Growth Hormone Physiology—Part 3," *Intensive Dietary Management*, https://idmprogram.com/fasting-and -growth-hormone-physiology-part-3/.

10. Fung, "Fasting and Growth Hormone Physiology—Part 3."

CHAPTER 5

1. Jason Fung, *The Obesity Code: Unlocking the Secrets of Weight Loss* (Vancouver: Greystone Books, 2016), 175–87.

2. Jason Fung explains the process with characteristic clarity in *The Obesity Code*, 78–88.

3. See "Carnivore Diet: Why Would It Work? What about Nutrients and Fiber?" *What I've Learned*, August 28, 2018, https://www.youtube.com /watch?v=isIw2AN-XU.

4. Pedro Carrera-Bastos, Maelan Fontes-Villalba, James H. O'Keefe, Staffan Lindeberg, Loren Cordain, "The Western Diet and Lifestyle and Diseases of Civilization," *Research Reports in Clinical Cardiology* 2 (2011): 15–35.

5. Liz Szabo, "Diabetes Rates Skyrocket in Kids and Teens," *USA Today*, May 3, 2014, https://www.usatoday.com/story/news/nation/2014/05/03 /diabetes-rises-in-kids/8604213/.

6. "Division of Diabetes Translation at a Glance," *National Center for Chronic Disease Prevent and Health Promotion,* https://www.cdc.gov /chronicdisease/resources/publications/aag/diabetes.htm.

CHAPTER 6

1. See the database maintained by the University of Sydney, which is quite detailed: http://www.glycemicindex.com/. See also the discussion in Fung, *The Obesity Code,* 176–78.
2. Gary Taubes, *Why We Get Fat: And What to Do About It* (New York: Knopf, 2010); Gary Taubes, *Good Calories, Bad Calories* (New York: Knopf, 2007); Nina Teicholz, *The Big Fat Surprise: Why Butter, Meat, and Cheese Belong in a Healthy Diet* (New York: Simon & Schuster, 2014).
3. Denise Minger, *Death by Food Pyramid* (Primal Nutrition, 2014).
4. Bret Scher, "Want a Healthier Heart? Eat a Steak," *Houston Chronicle,* September 19, 2018, https://www.houstonchronicle.com/opinion /outlook/article/want-a-healthier-heart-eat-a-steak-opinion-13239443 .php. The study he refers to is M. Dehghan et al., "Association of Fats and Carbohydrate Intake with Cardiovascular Disease and Mortality in 18 Countries from Five Continents (PURE): A Prospective Cohort Study," *Lancet,* November 4, 2017, https://www.ncbi.nlm.nih.gov /pubmed/28864332.
5. A recent and widely reported study claimed that low-carb, high-fat diets are unhealthy. But it was riddled with elementary errors. See the summary of its problems in Chris Kresser, "Will Low-Carb Kill You?" ChrisKresser.com, August 28, 2018, https://chriskresser.com/will-a-low -carb-diet-shorten-your-life/.
6. Liat Nachshon, Michael R. Goldberg, Arnon Elizur, Michael Y. Applebaum, Michael B. Levy, Yitzhak Katz, "Food Allergy to Previously Tolerated Foods," *Annals of Allergy, Asthma, and Immunology* 121, no. 1 (July 2018): 77–81.

CHAPTER 8

1. William Davis describes the symptoms, based on his clinical practice, in *Wheat Belly: Lose the Wheat, Lose the Weight, and Find Your Path Back to Health* (New York: Rodale Books, 2011).
2. G. L. Russo, "Dietary n-6 and n-3 Polyunsaturated Fatty Acids: From Biochemistry to Clinical Implications in Cardiovascular Prevention," *Biochemical Pharmacology* 77, no. 6 (2009): 937–46. See also https:// openheart.bmj.com/content/5/2/e000898.full.pdf.

3. See summary in Kris Gunnars, "Are Vegetable and Seed Oils Bad for Your Health?" *Healthline*, April 23, 2018, https://www.healthline.com /nutrition/are-vegetable-and-seed-oils-bad.

4. https://www.dietdoctor.com/low-carb/keto/recipes; https://www .ruled.me/best-keto-recipe-roundup-of-2014/; https://draxe.com/hub /keto-diet/keto-recipes/.

5. M. Yanina Pepino, Courtney D. Tiemann, Bruce W. Patterson, Burton M. Wice and Samuel Klein, "Sucralose Affects Glycemic and Hormonal Responses to an Oral Glucose Load," *Diabetes Care*, April 2013, http://care.diabetesjournals.org/content/36/9/2530.

6. M. Y. Pepino, C. Bourne, "Non-nutritive Sweeteners, Energy Balance, and Glucose Homeostasis," *Current Opinion in Clinical Nutrition & Metabolic Care* 14, no. 4 (July 2011): 391–95.

7. See the fuller discussion in "What Is the Keto Flu and How to Remedy It?" Ruled.me, https://www.ruled.me/keto-flu-remedy/.

8. See the discussion of recent studies and meta-analyses in Melinder Wenner Moyer, "It's Time to End the War on Salt," *Scientific American*, July 8, 2011, https://www.scientificamerican.com/article/its-time-to -end-the-war-on-salt/. See also Joseph Di Nicolantonio, *The Salt Fix: Why the Experts Got It All Wrong—and How Eating More Might Save Your Life* (New York: Harmony, 2017).

9. Jason Fung, "The Salt Scam," *Medium*, September 26, 2018, https:// medium.com/@drjasonfung/the-salt-scam-1973d73dccd.

10. From a huge 2010 meta-analysis: "During 5-23 y of follow-up of 347,747 subjects, 11,006 developed CHD or stroke. Intake of saturated fat was not associated with an increased risk of CHD, stroke, or CVD." P. W. Siri-Tarino, Q. Sun, F. B. Hu, and R. M. Krauss, "Meta-analysis of Prospective Cohort Studies Evaluating the Association of Saturated Fat with Cardiovascular Disease," *American Journal of Clinical Nutrition* 91, no. 3 (March 2013), https://www.ncbi.nlm.nih .gov/pubmed/20071648.

11. A 2018 media frenzy claimed just this. See Georgia Ede's response, "Latest Low Carb Study: All Politics, No Science," *Psychology Today*, September 18, 2018, https://www.psychologytoday.com/us/blog /diagnosis-diet/201809/latest-low-carb-study-all-politics-no-science.

12. Kimberly Leonard, "Here's What the Government Says You Should Eat," *US News & World Report*, January 7, 2016, https://www.usnews .com/news/articles/2016/01/07/new-nutrition-guidelines-meat-eggs -are-ok-to-eat-after-all-usda-says.

13. See https://www.headsuphealth.com/blog/self-tracking/low-carb-lab
-testing-part-8-the-cac-test-a-better-way-to-evaluate-cardiovascular-health
/. See also https://diabetesdietblog.com/2018/08/26/what-factors-are
-most-predictive-of-a-heart-attack/.

CHAPTER 9

1. St. Pope John Paul II, *Salvifici Doloris*, 1984, http://w2.vatican.va
/content/john-paul-ii/en/apost_letters/1984/documents/hf_jp-ii
_apl_11021984_salvifici-doloris.html.
2. Dave Armstrong, "Suffering with Christ Is a Biblical Teaching,"
National Catholic Register, March 27, 2018, http://www.ncregister.com
/blog/darmstrong/suffering-with-christ-is-a-biblical-teaching.
3. Matthew Becklo, "Priests on Long Island Undertake 25-Day
'Communal Penance of Fasting,'" *Aleteia*, September 1, 2018, https://
aleteia.org/2018/09/01/priests-on-long-island-undertake-25-day
-communal-penance-of-fasting/.
4. Paul VI, Apostolic Constitution *Paenitemini*, "On Fast and
Abstinence," February 17, 1966, http://w2.vatican.va/content/paul-vi
/en/apost_constitutions/documents/hf_p-vi_apc_19660217
_paenitemini.html.
5. Paul VI and John Paul II, *Fasting and Solidarity: Pontifical Messages for
Lent* (Pontifical Council Cor Unum, 1991), 17.

CHAPTER 10

1. See, for instance, Denise Winterman, "Breakfast, Lunch and Dinner:
Have We Always Eaten Them?" *BBC News Magazine*, November 14,
2012, https://www.bbc.com/news/magazine-20243692.
2. See Abigail Carroll, *Three Squares: The Invention of the American Meal*
(New York: Basic Books, 2013).

CHAPTER 11

1. Thomas Dubay, *Deep Conversion, Deep Prayer* (San Francisco: Ignatius
Press, 2006).
2. To fill out the day, the individual offices (fixed prayer times) became
longer and more elaborate. In monasteries, this allowed a one group
of monks to pray one hour, and then hand the duty off to another
group to pray the next hour.

     As with other practices, St. Benedict organized the texts of the
divine office in his rule. His great admonition, you might recall, was

"Orare est laborare, laborare est orare," that is, *"To pray is to work, to work is to pray."* The motto of the Benedictine order is simply *ora et labora*—work and pray.

3. The complete list of monastic prayers and their names is as follows. Only a few contemplative monasteries still keep all of these, and the first hour of the day has long since been suppressed:

Hour	Latin Name	English Name
During the Night	Matins	Readings
Sunrise	Lauds	Morning Prayer
First Hour of the Day	Prime	(suppressed)
Third Hour of the Day	Terce	Mid-morning Prayer
Sixth Hour of the Day	Sext	Midday Prayer
Ninth Hour of the Day	None	Mid-afternoon Prayer
As Evening Approaches	Vespers	Evening Prayer
Nightfall	Compline	Night Prayer

From "Liturgy of the Hours/Divine Office/Breviary, at: https://www.ewtn.com/expert/answers/breviary.htm.

4. Catholic priests and non-monastic religious orders pray at least the morning and evening prayers as part of their disciplines. Many orders have their own variations, but the most widely used form of the Divine Office since the Council of Trent is the Roman Office found in the common published volumes.

5. See "The Anglican Breviary: How to Recite the Office," Anglicanbreviary.net, https://www.anglicanbreviary.net/how-to-recite-the-office.

6. At http://www.peterkreeft.com/topics/time.htm.

CHAPTER 13

1. Anthony Esolen, "The Last Defender of Reason and the Human Body," *Crisis*, April 11, 2018, https://www.crisismagazine.com/2018/last-defender-reason-human-body.

2. Such as John Anthony McGuckin, *Westminster Handbook to Origen* (Philadelphia: Westminster John Knox Press, 2004).

3. The later Council of Constantinople, in AD 553, also condemned Origen's belief that everyone including the demons would be saved.

4. Caroline Walker Bynum, *Holy Feast and Holy Fast: The Religious Significance of Food to Medieval Women* (Berkeley, CA: University of California Press, 1987), 12.

5. Susan Mathews, "The Biblical Evidence on Fasting," *Diakonia* 24 (1991): 93–108.
6. Alexander Schmemann, *Great Lent: Journey to Pascha* (Crestwood, NY: St. Vladimir's Seminary Press, 1974), 28.

CHAPTER 15

1. Ori Hofmekler with Diana Holtzberg, *The Warrior Diet: How to Take Advantage of Undereating and Overeating* (St. Paul, MN: Dragon Door Publications, 1st edition, 2001).
2. See his videos and commentary at: https://fledgefitness.com/.

CHAPTER 16

1. Quoted in Alice Lady Lovat, *The Life of Saint Teresa* (St. Louis: B. Herder, 1912), 97.
2. Tiffany Greco, Thomas C. Glenn, David A. Hovda, and Mayumi L. Prins, "Ketogenic Diet Decreases Oxidative Stress and Improves Mitochondrial Complex Activity," *Journal of Cerebral Blood Flow Metabolism* 36, no. 9 (September 2016), https://www.ncbi.nlm.nih.gov/pmc/articles/PMC5012517/.
3. Emily Deans, "Your Brain on Ketones," *Psychology Today*, April 18, 2011, https://www.psychologytoday.com/us/blog/evolutionary-psychiatry/201104/your-brain-ketones.
4. Mark P. Mattson, Wenzhen Duan, Zhihong Guo, "Meal Size and Frequency Affect Neuronal Plasticity and Vulnerability to Disease: Cellular and Molecular Mechanisms," *Journal of Neurochemistry* 84, no. 3 (February 2003), https://onlinelibrary.wiley.com/doi/full/10.1046/j.1471-4159.2003.01586.x.
5. Manqi Wang, Qian Wang, and Matthew D. Whim, "Fasting Induces a Form of Autonomic Synaptic Plasticity that Prevents Hypoglycemia," *Proceedings of the National Academy of Sciences USA* 113, no. 21 (May 24, 2016), https://www.ncbi.nlm.nih.gov/pmc/articles/PMC4889352/.
6. Abdolhossein Bastani, Sadegh Rajabi, and Fatemeh Kianimarkani, "The Effect of Fasting During Ramadan on the Concentration of Serotonin, Dopamine, Brain-Derived Neurotrophic Factor and Nerve Growth Factor," *Neurology International* 9, no. 2 (June 23, 2017), https://www.ncbi.nlm.nih.gov/pmc/articles/PMC5505095/.
7. Clarisse A. Marotz and Amir Zarrinpar, "Treating Obesity and Metabolic Syndrome with Fecal Microbiota Transplantation," *Yale Journal of Biology and Medicine* 89, no. 3 (September 2016): 383–88. https://www.ncbi.nlm.nih.gov/pmc/articles/PMC5045147/.

8. See the NIH's "Human Microbiome Project" at: https://commonfund .nih.gov/hmp.
9. See references in Ruairi Robertson, "The Gut-Brain Connection: How It Works and the Role of Nutrition," *Healthline*, June 27, 2018, https:// www.healthline.com/nutrition/gut-brain-connection.
10. James H. Catterson, Mobina Khericha, Miranda C. Dyson, Alec J. Vincent, Rebecca Callard, Steven M. Haveron, Arjunan Rajasingam, Mumtaz Ahmad, and Linda Partridge, "Short-Term Intermittent Fasting Induces Long-Lasting Gut Health and TOR-Independent Lifespan Extension," *Current Biology* 28, no. 11 (June 4, 2018): 1714–24, https://www.ncbi.nlm.nih.gov/pmc/articles /PMC5988561/.
11. Craig Gustafson, "Alan Goldhamer, DC: Water Fasting—The Clinical Effectiveness of Rebooting Your Body," *Integrative Medicine: A Clinician's Journal* 13, no. 3 (June 2014), https://www.ncbi.nlm.nih .gov/pmc/articles/PMC4684131/.
12. Max Lugavere and Paul Grewal, *Genius Foods* (New York: Harper Wave, 2018); David Perlmutter, *Brain Maker: The Power of Gut Microbes to Heal and Protect Your Brain for Life* (New York: Little, Brown and Company, 2015).

CHAPTER 17

1. Michael Mosley, "The Power of Intermittent Fasting," *BBC News*, August 5, 2012, https://www.bbc.com/news/health-19112549.
2. He has also done studies on simpler organisms with very short life spans and discovered the same effect. He describes his research, and lays out the diet protocol, in *The Longevity Diet* (New York: Avery, 2018).
3. See a compilation of the key scientific studies online at: https:// l-nutra.com/scientific-articles/.
4. This is not the subject of this book. But for an accessible explanation of the flaws in many arguments a vegan or vegetarian diet offers increased longevity over an omnivorous diet, see Chris Kresser, "Do Vegetarians and Vegans Live Longer than Meat Eaters?" ChrisKresser.com, September 27, 2018, https://chriskresser.com/do -vegetarians-and-vegans-live-longer-than-meat-eaters/. The most obvious problem is the "healthy-user bias." Vegans and vegetarians tend to be more concerned with their health than the average omnivore. As a result, unless studies account for this variable, it will bias the results.

CHAPTER 19

1. For instance, it appears in *Ephraemi Rescriptus,* dated to the fifth century AD. But it's not in either *Codex Sinaiticus* or *Codex Vaticanus,* both of which date to the fourth century AD.

2. For instance, conservative evangelical D. A. Carson holds this view. See *Matthew: The Expositor's Bible Commentary* vol. 8 (Regency Reference Library, 1984), 392.

3. Michael Pakaluk, "Where Have All the Devils Gone?" *The Catholic Thing,* November 13, 2018, https://www.thecatholicthing.org/2018/11/13 /where-have-all-the-devils-gone/.

4. At Crossroads Initiative, https://www.crossroadsinitiative.com/media /articles/forty-days-lent/.

5. When Moses was with God on Mt. Sinai, he neither ate nor drank (Exodus 34:28). We can assume that God miraculously sustained him.

6. *Angelus,* St. Peter's Square (February 21, 2010), at: http://w2.vatican .va/content/benedict-xvi/en/angelus/2010/documents/hf_ben-xv i_ang_20100221.html.

7. See a detailed history, as well as a careful distinction between the historical facts and later embellishments, in Kevin Symonds, *Pope Leo XIII and the Prayer to St. Michael* (Preserving Christian Publications, 2nd edition, 2018).

CHAPTER 20

1. Kevin Loria, "The True Story of the Man Who Survived Without any Food for 382 Days," *Business Insider,* October 18, 2016, https://www .businessinsider.com.au/angus-barbieri-382-days-without-food -scotsman-fasting-starvation-obesity-2016-10.

2. See discussion of these experiments in Jason Fung, *The Obesity Code* (Vancouver: Greystone Books, 2016), 58.

3. Shubhroz Gill, Satchidananda Panda, "A Smartphone App Reveals Erratic Diurnal Eating Patterns in Humans that Can Be Modulated for Health Benefits," *Cell Metabolism,* September 24, 2015, https://www .cell.com/cell-metabolism/fulltext/S1550-4131%2815%2900462-3.

4. Michael Hobbes, "Everything You Know About Obesity Is Wrong," *Huffington Post,* September 19, 2018, https://highline.huffingtonpost.com /articles/en/everything-you-know-about-obesity-is-wrong/. See references.

5. J. D. Simkins, "A Staggering Number of Troops Are Fat and Tired, Report Says," *The Military Times,* October 3, 2018, https://www.militarytimes .com/off-duty/military-culture/2018/10/03/a-staggering-number-of -troops-are-fat-and-tired-report-says/.

6. Fung, *The Obesity Code*, 78.

7. See Megan Ramos, "What Is Fat Fasting and When Should You Do It?" *Intensive Dietary Management*, https://idmprogram.com/what-is-fat -fasting-and-when-should-you-do-it/.

8. Frank Q. Muttall, Rami M. Almokayyad, Mary C. Gannon, "Comparison of a Carbohydrate-Free Diet vs. Fasting on Plasma Glucose, Insulin and Glucagon in Type 2 Diabetes," *Metabolism* 64, no. 2 (February 2015): 253–62.

9. Are dietary guidelines proof of a vast conspiracy between government and Big Food to get everyone addicted to sugar and fake food when the universe meant for us to eat only whole plants? A dozen documentaries on Netflix say yes. Sort of. And even fine books by scientists such as Robert Lustig, such as *Fat Chance* and *The Hacking of the American Mind*, go in for conspiracies.

   There's a better explanation, obvious to anyone who has studied the history and philosophy of science and Public Choice and behavioral economics. People respond to incentives. As a result, large companies in a cozy relationship with government may do harmful things, even if they think they're trying to help. Scientists funded by the corn or sugar lobby likely suffer from confirmation bias and theory-induced blindness. So, they may really believe the results of their experiments just happen to support the corn or sugar lobby. Government agencies may harm or even kill people, without trying, let alone wanting, to do so. We can explain these things without invoking conspiracies. Indeed, the conspiratorial tone in the alt diet community slows its wider acceptance.

CHAPTER 21

1. See, for instance, Belinda S. Lennerz, Anna Barton, Richard K. Bernstein, R. David Dikeman, Carrie Diulus, Sarah Hallberg, Erinn T. Rhodes, Cara B. Ebbeling, Eric C. Westman, William S. Yancy Jr., David S. Ludwig, "Management of Type 1 Diabetes with a Very Low-Carbohydrate Diet," *Pediatrics* 141, no. 6 (June 2018), http://pediatrics .aappublications.org/content/pediatrics/141/6/e20173349.full.pdf.

2. Matteo Fumagalli et al., "Greenland Inuit Show Genetics Signatures of Diet and Climate Adaptation," *Science* 349, no. 6254 (September 18, 2015): 1343–47.

3. Pedro Carrera-Bastos, Maelan Fontes-Villalba, James H O'Keefe, Staffan Lindeberg, Loren Cordain, "The Western Diet and Lifestyle and Diseases of Civilization," *Research Reports in Clinical Cardiology* 2 (March 9, 2011),

https://www.dovepress.com/the-western-diet-and-lifestyle-and
-diseases-of-civilization-peer-reviewed-article-RRCC.

4. B. Chiofalo et al., "Fasting as Possible Complementary Approach for
   Polycystic Ovary Syndrome: Hope or Hype?" *Medical Hypotheses* 105
   (August 2017): 1–3.

5. Dale Bredesen, *The End of Alzheimer's* (New York: Avery, 2017); Amy
   Berger, *The Alzheimer's Antidote* (White River Junction, VT: Chelsea
   Green Publishing, 2017).

6. J. M. Freeman, E. P. Vining, "Seizures Decrease Rapidly After Fasting:
   Preliminary Studies of the Ketogenic Diet," *Archives of Pediatric &
   Adolescent Medicine* 153, no. 9 (1999), 946–49.

7. See discussion of ketogenic diets at the Epilepsy Foundation, at:
   https://www.epilepsy.com/learn/treating-seizures-and-epilepsy
   /dietary-therapies/ketogenic-diet.

8. Adam L. Hartman, James E. Rubenstein, and Eric H. Kossoff,
   "Intermittent Fasting: A 'New' Historical Strategy for Controlling
   Seizures?" *Epilepsy Research* 104, no. 3 (May 2013): 275–79.

9. Patients on a low-fat, high carb diet improved in their motor skills,
   but not their non-motor skills. Matthew C. L. Phillips et al., "Low-Fat
   Versus Ketogenic Diet in Parkinson's Disease: A Pilot Randomized
   Controlled Trial," *Movement Disorders* 33, no. 8 (August 2018), https://
   onlinelibrary.wiley.com/doi/abs/10.1002/mds.27390.

10. Matthew G. Vander Heiden, Lewis C. Cantley, and Craig B.
    Thompson, "Understanding the Warburg Effect: The Metabolic
    Requirements of Cell Proliferation," *Science* (May 22, 2009): 1029–33.

11. As Warburg put it: "Cancer, above all other diseases, has countless
    secondary causes. But, even for cancer, there is only one prime
    cause. Summarized in a few words, the prime cause of cancer is the
    replacement of the respiration of oxygen in normal body cells by a
    fermentation of sugar."

12. Thomas Seyfried, *Cancer as a Metabolic Disease: On the Origin,
    Management, and Prevention of Cancer* (New York: Wiley, 2012).
    See also Travis Kristofferson, *Tripping over the Truth* (White River
    Junction, VT: Chelsea Green Publishing, 2017.)

13. In mouse studies, researchers often refer to STS (short-term starvation)
    rather than fasting. See, for instance, L. Raffaghello, C. Lee, F. M.
    Safdie, M. Wei, F. Madia, G. Bianchi, V. D. Longo, "Starvation-
    Dependent Differential Stress Resistance Protects Normal but Not
    Cancer Cells Against High-Dose Chemotherapy," *Proceedings of the
    National Academic of Sciences USA* 105 (2008): 8215–20; C. Lee et al.,

"Fasting Cycles Retard Growth of Tumors and Sensitize a Range of Cancer Cell Types to Chemotherapy," *Science Translational Medicine* 4 (2012): 124–27; F. Safdie et al., "Fasting Enhances the Response of Glioma to Chemo- and Radiotherapy," *PLOS One* 7 (2012), https://journals.plos.org/plosone/article?id=10.1371/journal.pone.0044603.

14. A. M. Poff, C. Ari, P. Arnold, T. N. Seyfried, and D. P. D'Agostino, "Ketone Supplementation Decreases Tumor Cell Viability and Prolongs Survival of Mice with Metastatic Cancer," *International Journal of Cancer* 135, no. 7 (October 2014): 1711–20, https://www.ncbi.nlm.nih.gov/pmc/articles/PMC4235292/.

15. F. M. Safdie, T. Dorff, D. Quinn, L. Fontana, M. Wei, C. Lee, P. Cohen, V. D. Longo, "Fasting and Cancer Treatment in Humans: A Case Series Report," *Aging* 1 (2009): 988–1007.

16. Alessio Nencioni, Irene Caffa, Salvatore Cortellino, and Valter D. Longo, "Fasting and Cancer: Molecular Mechanisms and Clinical Application," *Nature Reviews Cancer* 18 (2018): 707–19.

17. Yun-Hee Youm et al., "The Ketone Metabolite β-Hydroxybutyrate Blocks Nlrp3 Inflammasome–Mediated Inflammatory Disease," *Nature Medicine* 21 (2015): 263–69.

18. L. Fontana and L. Partridge, "Promoting Health and Longevity Through Diet: From Model Organisms to Humans," *Cell* 161, no. 1 (March 26, 2015): 106–18.

19. Quoted in Karen Feldscher, "In Pursuit of Healthy Aging," *The Harvard Gazette*, November 3, 2017, https://news.harvard.edu/gazette/story/2017/11/intermittent-fasting-may-be-center-of-increasing-lifespan/.

20. This may be new information to you. In fact, it's new information for everyone. It was just in 2016 that Yoshinori Ohsumi won the Nobel prize for medicine for his research on autophagy.

21. mTOR is shorthand for "mammalian target of rapamycin." Jason Fung provides more details in "Fasting and Autophagy—mTOR/Autophagy 1," *Intensive Dietary Management*, at: https://idmprogram.com/fasting-and-autophagy-mtor-autophagy-1/.

22. I'm paraphrasing, with some tweaks, the famous "hallmarks of cancer" described by Douglas Hanahan and Robert A. Weinberg, which they updated and supplemented in "Hallmarks of Cancer: The Next Generation," *Cell* 144, no. 5 (March 4, 2011): 646–74.

23. Like other cells, cancer cells convert nutrients into a chemical form of energy called ATP (adenosine triphosphate). But cancer cells have fewer ways of producing ATP compared to healthy cells.

24. This is yet another topic on which far more research is needed. For recent research, see article and references in Mohammad Derakhshan, Reza Derakhshan, "Fasting and Apoptosis: A Mini Review," *Journal of Fasting and Health* 3, no. 5 (2015): 166–68, http://jnfh.mums.ac.ir/article_6314_c25aae79680a5a68a69d6c21dc8a99fa.pdf.

25. Kelly McGonigal, *The Upside of Stress: How Stress Is Good for You, and How to Get Good at It* (New York: Avery, 2nd edition, 2015); Andrew Bernstein offers practical strategies for changing how you think about and experience stress in *The Myth of Stress* (New York: Atria Books, 2010).

CHAPTER 23

1. Josemaría Escrivá de Balaguer, *The Way* (New York: Scepter, 1953), 179.
2. See discussion of studies in Alysse ElHage, "The Power of Prayer in Families," *Institute for Family Studies*, September 13, 2018, https://ifstudies.org/blog/the-power-of-prayer-for-families.
3. Subjects in one small clinical trial on the "Daniel Fast" improved "several risk factors for metabolic and cardiovascular disease." Richard J. Bloomer, Mohammad M. Kabir, Robert E. Canale, John F. Trepanowski, Kate E. Marshall, Tyler M. Farney, and Kelley G. Hammond, "Effect of a 21 Day Daniel Fast on Metabolic and Cardiovascular Disease Risk Factors in Men and Women," *Lipids in Health and Disease* 9 (2010), https://www.ncbi.nlm.nih.gov/pmc/articles/PMC2941756/.
4. John Piper, *A Hunger for God: Desiring God Through Fasting and Prayer* (Wheaton, IL: Crossway, Redesign edition, 2013).
5. Jentezen Franklin, *Fasting: Opening the Door to a Deeper, More Intimate, More Powerful Relationship with God* (Nashville: Charisma House, 2007).
6. The calendars of East and West differ a bit, unfortunately. But most Latin Catholic and Protestant churches follow a Western calendar, so feasts and fasts will fall on the same days for both.

CHAPTER 24

1. Robert Morlino, "Bishop Robert C. Morlino's Letter to the Faithful Regarding the Ongoing Sexual Abuse Crisis in the Church," *Diocese of Madison Catholic Herald*, August 18, 2018, http://www.madisoncatholicherald.org/bishopsletters/7730-letter-scandal.html.
2. Michael Pakaluk, "Easter Is Fundamentally Apostolic," *The Catholic Thing*, April 3, 2018, https://www.thecatholicthing.org/2018/04/03/easter-is-fundamentally-apostolic/.

3. Another fast common in the Christian tradition, and still retained in Eastern churches, is the Apostles' Fast. It starts after Pentecost, in imitation of the apostles who fasted and prayed after the Pentecost miracle in the book of Acts. It is less strict than Lent. Eastern Rite and Orthodox Christians abstain from meat and dairy during this time. It varies in length, because Easter and Pentecost move around the calendar, but it always ends with the Feasts of St. Peter and Paul on June 29.

CHAPTER 25

1. Bill Bright, "How Long and What Type of Fast Is Right for You," *CRU*, https://www.cru.org/us/en/train-and-grow/spiritual-growth/fasting/personal-guide-to-fasting.4.html.
2. Bill Bright, *The Coming Revival: America's Call to Fast, Pray, and Seek God's Face* (Orlando, FL: New Life Publications, 1995).
3. Laurie Goodstein, "In Hope of Spiritual Revival, a Call to Fast," *New York Times*, February 9, 1998, https://www.nytimes.com/1998/02/08/us/in-hope-of-spiritual-revival-a-call-to-fast.html.
4. Bill Bright, "While You Fast," https://www.cru.org/us/en/train-and-grow/spiritual-growth/fasting/7-steps-to-fasting.3.html.
5. K. Y. Ho, J. D. Veldhuis, R. Furlanetto, W. S. Evans, K. G. Alberti, and M. O. Thorner, "Fasting Enhances Growth Hormone Secretion and Amplifies the Complex Rhythms of Growth Hormone Secretion in Man," *Journal of Clinical Investigation* 81, no. 4 (April 1988): 968–75. https://www.ncbi.nlm.nih.gov/pmc/articles/PMC329619/.
6. See information at their website: https://www.healthpromoting.com/. Two scientific articles provide evidence that water-only fasts are useful in treating high blood pressure: Alan Goldhamer, Douglas Lisle, Banoo Parpia, Scott V. Anderson, and T. Colin Campbell, "Medically Supervised Water-Only Fasting in the Treatment of Hypertension," *Journal of Manipulative and Physiological Therapeutics* 24, no. 5 (June 2001), https://www.scribd.com/doc/32727377/medically-supervised-water-only-fasting-in-the-treatment-of-hypertension. Alan C. Goldhamer, Douglas J. Lisle, Peter Sultana, Scott V. Anderson, Banoo Parpia, Barry Hughes, and T. Colin Campbell, "Medically Supervised Water-Only Fasting in the Treatment of Borderline Hypertension," *The Journal of Alternative and Complementary Medicine* 8, no. 5 (2002): 643–50, https://www.scribd.com/document/32727203/medically-supervised-water-only-fasting-in-the-treatment-of-borderline-hypertension.

7. Markham Heid, "Why Fasting Diets Are About to Get More Extreme," *Medium*, October 11, 2018, https://medium.com/s/the-nuance/why -fasting-diets-of-the-future-may-be-even-more-extreme-bf8db9befa70.
8. Megan Ramos, "What Is Fat Fasting and When Should You Do It?" *Intensive Dietary Management*, https://idmprogram.com/what-is-fat -fasting-and-when-should-you-do-it/.

CHAPTER 26
1. Richard Dawkins, *The Blind Watchmaker* (New York: W. W. Norton, 1986).
2. Quoted in Henry Margenau and Roy Abraham Varghese, editors, *Cosmos, Bios, Theos* (La Salle, IL: Open Court, 1992), 83.
3. The full quote is: "Because there is a law such as gravity, the universe can and will create itself from nothing. Spontaneous creation is the reason there is something rather than nothing, why the universe exists, why we exist." Stephen Hawking and Leonard Mlodinow, *The Grand Design* (New York: Bantam, 2010). I discuss the problems with Hawking's claim in Jay Richards, "Did Physics Kill God?" *The American*, November 3, 2010, http://www.aei.org/publication/did-physics-kill-god/.
4. For an excellent explanation of the scientific evidence for the power and limits of natural selection and random variation, see Michael Behe, *The Edge of Evolution: The Search for the Limits of Darwinism* (New York: The Free Press, 2008).
5. The documentary *Expelled* details multiple such cases of their jackbooted tactics, and I am familiar with many more. In this sort of atmosphere, most with doubts about Darwinism learn to keep their mouths shut and their heads down. A few brave scientists—usually ones with tenure and who are nearing retirement—have stuck their necks out by signing a Dissent from Darwin statement, now with more than a thousand signatures.
6. See Michael J. Behe, *Darwin Devolves: The News About DNA that Challenges Evolution* (San Francisco: HarperOne, 2019), 256.
7. Douglas Axe, *Undeniable: How Biology Confirms Our Intuition that Life Is Designed* (San Francisco: HarperOne, 2016).
8. Jared Diamond, "The Worst Mistake in the History of the Human Race," *Discover*, May 1, 1999, http://discovermagazine.com/1987 /may/02-the-worst-mistake-in-the-history-of-the-human-race.

CHAPTER 27
1. https://idmprogram.com/my-single-best-weight-loss-tip/.
2. Michael Pollan, *In Defense of Food: An Eater's Manifesto* (New York:

Penguin Books, 2008). He considers this a summary of everything he has learned about food and eating.

3. From Robb Wolf, *Wired to Eat: Turn Off Craving, Rewire Your Appetite for Weight Loss, and Determine the Foods that Work for You* (New York: Harmony, 2017).

4. Cara B. Ebbeling et al., "Effects of a Low Carbohydrate Diet on Energy Expenditure During Weight Loss Maintenance: Randomized Trial," *BMJ* 363 (2018), https://www.bmj.com/content/363/bmj.k4583.

CHAPTER 28

1. Roman Catholic canon law recognizes three types of events. The most important are solemnities, which mark the most important facts of salvation history, such as Christ's incarnation and resurrection. Second are feasts, which include Sundays; third are memorials. These are all celebrations, however, and so all qualify broadly as feasts as I'm using the term.

2. Josef Pieper, *In Tune with the World: A Theory of Festivity* (South Bend, IN: St. Augustine's Press, 1999), 3. The English words "feast," "festival," and "festive" derive from the German words *Fest* and *Feier*, which are the words Pieper uses, since he wrote the book in German.

3. Pieper, 3–4.

4. See description by C. Danko, "Once Upon a Time, When Christmas Was Banned," *A Puritan Mind*, http://www.apuritansmind.com /puritan-worship/christmas-and-the-regulative-principle/once -upon-a-time-when-christmas-was-banned-by-c-danko/; and Remy Melina, "The Surprising Truth: Christians Once Banned Christmas," *LiveScience*, December 14, 2010, https://www.livescience.com/32891 -why-was-christmas-banned-in-america-.html.

5. Robb Wolf argues forcefully in *Wired to Eat* that we should not treat even regular eating days as if they are "cheat days."

6. See Michael Pollan, *In Defense of Food: An Eater's Manifesto* (New York: Penguin Books, 2008).

7. Leon Kass, *The Hungry Soul: Eating and the Perfecting of Our Nature* (Chicago: University of Chicago Press), 134.

CONCLUSION

1. See Benjamin Wiker and Jonathan Witt, *A Meaningful World: How the Arts and Sciences Reveal the Genius of Nature* (Downers Grove, IL: InterVarsity Press Academic, 2006).

2. Catherine R. Marinac, "Prolonged Nightly Fasting and Breast Cancer

Risk: Findings from NHANES (2009–2010)," *Cancer Epidemiology, Biomarkers & Prevention* 24, no. 5 (May 2015): 783–89, https://www.ncbi.nlm.nih.gov/pmc/articles/PMC4417458/.

3. P. D. Mangan, "Lower Insulin Means Greater Fat Loss," *Medium*, August 12, 2016, https://medium.com/the-mission/the-sweet-spot-for-intermittent-fasting-9aae12a2158c.

4. I'm referring to the Real Presence rather than a detailed concept of transubstantiation per se, which Thomas Aquinas developed in the thirteenth century as a way to understand the Real Presence. The Real Presence is the belief that in some mysterious way, in the Eucharist, what appears as bread and wine really becomes the body and blood of Christ. Indeed, this belief was one of the basic markers of orthodoxy for most of Christian history.

5. John Paul II, General Audience, February 20, 1980, http://w2.vatican.va/content/john-paul-ii/en/audiences/1980/documents/hf_jp-ii_aud_19800220.html.

6. In his poem "On Liberty," section 8, Percy Bysshe Shelley mourns the loss of the pre-Christian West of Greece and Rome, which he considers Christianity to have spoiled: "The Galilean serpent forth did creep / And made thy world an undistinguishable heap."

7. John Piper, *A Hunger for God: Desiring God Through Fasting and Prayer* (Wheaton, IL: Crossway, Redesign edition, 2013).

8. Scott Hahn, *The Lamb's Supper: The Mass as Heaven on Earth* (New York: Image, 1999). See also Scott Hahn, *The Fourth Cup: Unveiling the Mystery of the Last Supper* (New York: Image, 2018).

APPENDIX 3

1. This term was coined by Jeff Volek and Stephen Phinney in *The Art and Science of Low Carbohydrate Living*.

2. For more on this and other problems, see Bjarte Bakke, "Why You're Not in Ketosis," *Diet Doctor*, May 16, 2017, https://www.dietdoctor.com/why-youre-not-in-ketosis.

3. See https://www.dietdoctor.com/low-carb/fasting-blood-glucose-higher.

4. https://optimisingnutrition.com/2015/07/20/the-glucose-ketone-relationship/.

INDEX

Scripture citations are listed under "Bible."